NEW FRONTIERS IN PEDIATRIC TRAUMATIC BRAIN INJURY

New Frontiers in Pediatric Traumatic Brain Injury provides an evidence base for clinical practice specific to traumatic brain injury (TBI) sustained during childhood, with a focus on functional outcomes. It utilizes a biological-psychosocial conceptual framework consistent with the International Classification of Functioning, Disability and Health, which highlights that biological, psychological, and social factors all play a role in disease and children's recovery from acquired brain injury. With its clinical perspective, it incorporates current and past research and evidence regarding advances that have occurred in outcomes, predictors, medical technology, and rehabilitation post-TBI.

This book is a great resource for established and new clinicians and researchers, graduate students, and postdoctoral fellows who work in the field of pediatric TBI, including psychologists, neuropsychologists, pediatricians, and psychiatrists.

Dr. Cathy Catroppa is an educational and developmental psychologist, a Research Fellow of the Murdoch Childrens Research Institute (MCRI), Royal Children's Hospital (RCH) in Melbourne, Australia, and Associate Professor in the Departments of Psychological Sciences and Paediatrics, University of Melbourne.

Dr. Vicki Anderson is Director of Psychology at the Royal Children's Hospital in Melbourne, Australia, Director of Critical Care and Neurosciences Research at the Murdoch Childrens Research Institute and Professor of Pediatrics and Psychology at the University of Melbourne.

Dr. Miriam Helen Beauchamp is Associate Professor in the Department of Psychology, University of Montreal and Researcher at the St. Justine Hospital Research Centre, where she leads the ABCs Developmental Neuropsychology Laboratory.

Dr. Keith Owen Yeates is Professor of Psychology, University of Calgary, where he is a member of the Alberta Children's Hospital Research Institute and Hotchkiss Brain Institute.

American Academy of Clinical Neuropsychology/ Routledge Continuing Education Book Series

Series Editors: Joel E. Morgan and Jerry J. Sweet

AACN/Routledge Continuing Education Series publishes authored and edited volumes containing a blend of cutting-edge primary research and practical/professional material for clinicians, researchers, and students of clinical neuropsychology and clinical psychology.

Each volume is written or edited by leading scholars in the field and is specifically designed to assist readers in advancing their relevant research or professional activities in clinical neuropsychology. Volumes in this series have been selected by the series editors because they provide one or more of the following: overview of a core or emerging area of concern to clinical neuropsychologists; in-depth examination of a specific area of research or practice in clinical neuropsychology; update of a neglected or controversial clinical application; information pertaining to relevance of a new interdisciplinary discovery/technique to neuropsychological function; or current ethical matters and other professional considerations in the application of new knowledge or methods to the understanding of neuropsychological functions.

AACN Online System

Any licensed psychologist who reads one of the books in the AACN/Routledge series will be able to earn CE credits by reading designated books and completing an online quiz.

To Receive Online Credit

- Read one of the CE-designated books in its entirety
- Access the CE quiz online at the AACN website (www.theaacn.org)
- Register for the specific book for which you wish to receive CE credit, and
- Complete all questions on the quiz.

The estimated time to read the book and complete the related quiz is determined by the length of each book, which also determines the number of possible credits.

The cost of CE credits is noted on the AACN website, and is reduced for AACN members and affiliates. Credit will be awarded to individuals scoring 80% or higher on the quiz. Participants will receive an immediate confirmation of credits earned by email.

CE Accreditation Statement

AACN is approved by the American Psychological Association to sponsor continuing education for psychologists. AACN maintains responsibility for this program and its content.

For more information on new and forthcoming titles in the Series and for instructions on how to take the accompanying online CE tests, please visit **www.theaacn.org** or **www.routledge.com/series/AACN**

NEW FRONTIERS IN PEDIATRIC TRAUMATIC BRAIN INJURY

An Evidence Base for Clinical Practice

Cathy Catroppa, Vicki Anderson,
Miriam H. Beauchamp,
and Keith Owen Yeates

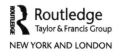

Routledge
Taylor & Francis Group

NEW YORK AND LONDON

First published 2016
by Routledge
711 Third Avenue, New York, NY 10017

and by Routledge
2 Park Square, Milton Park, Abingdon, Oxon, OX14 4RN

Routledge is an imprint of the Taylor & Francis Group, an informa business

Library of Congress Cataloging-in-Publication Data
Names: Catroppa, Cathy, author. | Anderson, Vicki, 1958– , author. |
    Beauchamp, Miriam H., author. | Yeates, Keith Owen, author.
Title: New frontiers in pediatric traumatic brain injury : an evidence base
    for clinical practice / Cathy Catroppa, Vicki Anderson, Miriam H.
    Beauchamp, and Keith Owen Yeates.
Description: New York, NY : Routledge, 2016. | Includes bibliographical
    references and index.
Identifiers: LCCN 2015029452 | ISBN 9781848728769 (hb : alk. paper) |
    ISBN 9781848726550 (pb : alk. paper) | ISBN 9780203868621 (eb)
Subjects: | MESH: Brain Injuries. | Child. | Evidence-Based Medicine. |
    Social Behavior.
Classification: LCC RJ496.B7 | NLM WS 340 | DDC
    617.4/81044083—dc23
LC record available at http://lccn.loc.gov/2015029452

ISBN: 978-1-84872-876-9 (hbk)
ISBN: 978-1-84872-655-0 (pbk)
ISBN: 978-0-203-86862-1 (ebk)

Typeset in Bembo
by Apex CoVantage, LLC

CONTENTS

SECTION III
Evidence-Based Outcomes and Their Predictors Following Child TBI

SECTION IV
Rehabilitation/Intervention

ABOUT THE AUTHORS

Dr. Cathy Catroppa is an educational and developmental psychologist, a Research Fellow of the Murdoch Childrens Research Institute (MCRI), Royal Children's Hospital (RCH) in Melbourne, Australia, and Associate Professor in the Departments of Psychological Sciences and Paediatrics, University of Melbourne. Her work has focused on the coordination of a large-scale research program examining acute and long-term outcomes following pediatric TBI. She has now also placed an emphasis on developing and piloting intervention programs aimed at preventing and/or reducing impairments following pediatric TBI. She has over 100 publications in peer-reviewed journals.

Dr. Vicki Anderson is Director of Psychology at the Royal Children's Hospital in Melbourne, Australia, Director of Critical Care and Neurosciences Research at the Murdoch Childrens Research Institute, and Professor of Pediatrics and Psychology at the University of Melbourne. She also established the Centre for Child Neuropsychological Studies. She has served on the board of governors of the International Neuropsychological Society and was president of the Australian Society for the Study of Brain Impairment. Her work focuses on the outcomes of developmental and acquired brain disorders in children, particularly TBI. She has over 200 publications in peer-reviewed journals.

Dr. Miriam Helen Beauchamp is Associate Professor in the Department of Psychology at the University of Montreal and a researcher at the St. Justine Hospital Research Centre, where she leads the ABCs Developmental Neuropsychology Laboratory. She is also Adjunct Professor in the Department of Neurology and Neurosurgery at McGill University. In 2015, she was awarded the International Neuropsychological Society Early Career Award in recognition for her work in the field of pediatric traumatic brain injury. She has training in both clinical neuropsychology and neuroscience, and her work focuses on using multi-modal approaches to study cognitive and social development in normative populations and in children and adolescents with brain injury.

Dr. Keith Owen Yeates is Professor of Psychology at the University of Calgary, where he is a member of the Alberta Children's Hospital Research Institute and Hotchkiss Brain Institute. He has served as president of the Society of Clinical Neuropsychology of the American Psychological Association and president of the Association for Postdoctoral Programs in Clinical Neuropsychology. He has published extensively in the area of childhood brain injury, with interests including acquired and developmental brain disorders, acute and long-term outcomes, predictors of outcome, and the neural substrates of cognitive function. He has authored over 150 peer-reviewed journal articles and 40 book chapters, and he has edited 4 books.

ACKNOWLEDGMENTS

Cathy Catroppa would like to thank all the authors who contributed to this book for sharing their expertise and presenting up-to-date information in the area of pediatric traumatic brain injury. She would also like to thank Psychology Press for their continual encouragement and guidance. She greatly appreciates the referencing and editing assistance of Kate Anderson, Celia Godfrey, and Phoebe Kho. A special thank you to all the children and families who take part in our clinical research. Without all of these contributions, this book would not have been possible.

PREFACE

The primary aim of *New Frontiers in Pediatric Traumatic Brain Injury: An Evidence Base for Clinical Practice* is to provide an evidence base for clinical practice specific to traumatic brain injury (TBI) sustained during childhood, with a focus on functional outcomes. The need for an evidence base to guide clinical practice highlights the importance of the scientist-practitioner model, in which research evidence and the application of this knowledge by the practitioner to clinical practice are paramount to improving the effectiveness of health care. A secondary aim of this text is to incorporate a bio–psycho-social conceptual framework when establishing such an evidence base. The bio-psycho-social model suggests that biological factors (e.g., an underlying disruption in the body), psychological factors (e.g., emotional difficulties), and social factors (e.g., family environment) all play a role in disease and in recovery from disease. Consistent with this model, the International Classification of Functioning, Disability and Health (ICF) framework, endorsed in 2001 and used to measure health and disability, also recognizes the importance of the disorder/disease, the role of personal/psychological factors, and the contribution of environmental factors and their combined influence on the quality of life of the individual. In 2010, the ICF established the same categories to address outcomes following traumatic brain injury.

In the 1980s, Michael Rutter and colleagues investigated aspects of child TBI (e.g., cognitive, behavioral, psychiatric, and educational outcomes), keeping in mind biological, psychological, and social influences and their effect on outcome. Since the 1990s, research on child TBI has grown substantially. Of particular importance is the methodological and conceptual progress that has been made, from case study material and small sample sizes, to larger case-control studies, to prospective longitudinal research, to the establishment of multi-disciplinary work with the inclusion of medical, neuropsychological, allied health, and imaging components, and to the development of intervention programs for the remediation of sequelae post-TBI.

In an attempt to incorporate this rich knowledge base about child TBI, and unlike previous books that have focused on a particular aspect of child TBI, this text offers the reader a comprehensive outlook on the characteristics and repercussions of these early injuries, from the time of the accident and throughout the life span. It adopts a clinical perspective, incorporating current and past research and evidence regarding advances in areas such as outcomes, predictors, medical technology, and rehabilitation post-TBI. Given the breadth of information—theoretical, clinical, and evidence-based—we believe the text will appeal to a wide range of health professionals, researchers, and educators.

1

INTRODUCTION

Traumatic brain injury (TBI) is a major public health problem among children and adolescents. In fact, TBI represents the leading cause of morbidity and mortality in children and adolescents (Anderson, Catroppa, Morse, Haritou, & Rosenfeld, 2005a) in developed nations. Perhaps because of the significant ongoing costs to not only survivors of TBI, but also their family and the community more generally, interest in TBI has exploded in the past few decades. This interest has led to advances in acute medical treatments. Recent research has focused on, among other things, the reduction of preventable secondary brain insult via faster medical response, potentially predictive biomarkers for early detection of injury, and interventions such as hypothermia. Advances in brain imaging have assisted in early diagnosis of TBI and helped guide appropriate treatment, with current high-resolution imaging enabling the identification of even subtle brain damage in the context of mild TBI. Evidence from both structural and functional imaging technologies increasingly shows common patterns of brain pathology resulting from pediatric TBI, both macroscopic and microscopic, and changes that occur over time in response to damage to the developing brain.

Researchers have also been reasonably successful in describing the longer-term consequences of child TBI, especially more serious injuries. The natural history of child TBI has been studied extensively, and we now have a working understanding of the acute and long-term effects of injury for the child and family. The next step is to translate empirical findings into clinically relevant information in order to develop, improve, and appropriately target evidence-based approaches to facilitate better outcomes for the child and family.

There are, however, several very real obstacles, many of them specific to this particular population. To begin, child TBI has not attracted the public attention that other childhood disorders receive, possibly because the consequences of TBI are often "masked," with most children appearing "normal" after injury, despite suffering from functionally significant impairments. An additional complication is that children who suffer TBI are not representative of the healthy population; they are more likely to have pre-existing behavioral and learning problems, as well as social disadvantages (Taylor & Alden, 1997). These factors may negatively affect recovery, as well as confound our ability to determine which post-injury difficulties are due to TBI and which might have predated the injury.

This book aims to contribute to knowledge about child TBI and its relevance to clinical practice. We have chosen to place particular emphasis on understanding of children's post-injury function, recovery, and outcomes, as well as factors that help predict recovery at the individual level. In order to achieve this goal, the book is divided into four sections: i) epidemiology and physiology of child TBI; ii) developmentally appropriate measurement and assessment considerations; iii) a comprehensive description of the functional consequences of child TBI and the factors that contribute to them; and iv) a review of evidence-based management and treatment approaches.

Epidemiology and Pathophysiology of Child TBI

Epidemiological data demonstrate that one in every 20 emergency department presentations at pediatric hospitals is for a TBI, making TBI more common than burns or poisonings. In the context of infancy, childhood, and adolescence, such injuries represent a common interruption to normal development, with population estimates ranging from 200 to over 500 per 100,000 a year and with well-established variations across age and gender (Crowe, Babl, Anderson, & Catroppa, 2009; Langlois, Rutland-Brown, & Thomas, 2006). Fortunately, the majority of TBIs sustained by children and adolescents are mild, typically with few long-term consequences; however, a significant proportion of children will experience a range of residual and persisting physical, cognitive, educational, functional, social, and emotional consequences. These children and adolescents will require lifelong health care across a range of disciplines, leading to a significant social and economic burden for the children's families and for the community more broadly (Cassidy, Carroll, Peloso, Borg, et al., 2004).

Further, research has established that the mechanisms of injury often vary with developmental stage. For example, injuries due to child abuse are almost exclusive to infants, whereas in preschool children, the majority of injuries occur as a result of falls from furniture or play equipment. These early injuries are likely to be linked closely to environmental factors, such as family dysfunction and social disadvantage. In contrast, in older children, injuries are more likely to be due to sporting or motor vehicle accidents and can be more directly associated with the child's own actions and behavior. In light of these epidemiological data, communities are beginning to take steps to educate people about and prevent TBI. For example, in some countries, helmets have been mandated for bicycle riders and participants in certain contact sports.

Developmental Considerations

In recent decades, researchers and clinicians working with children with TBI have become aware that children are not simply "little adults" and that injuries to the immature brain cannot be understood or treated in the same manner as adult injuries. In fact, evidence increasingly indicates that age and skill attainment at the time of injury are important considerations in assessing the impact for neural networks and the likelihood of recovery. Although the field of child TBI is largely guided by science and practice in adult TBI, developmental and contextual issues need to be taken into account at all stages of recovery and treatment. Until relatively recently, our understanding of recovery and outcomes following child TBI lagged behind that for adults. This is changing. Research in child TBI has grown enormously and now has more solid foundations. Key principles have been established, some of which are consistent with the adult literature, such as the predictive value of injury severity (Anderson, Morse, Catroppa, Haritou, & Rosenfeld, 2004; Taylor, Swartwout, Yeates, Walz, et al., 2008). Others are child-specific—for example, the unique mechanics and characteristic pathology of inflicted injury in children (Coats & Margulies, 2006; Prange & Margulies, 2002)—or reflect the importance of developmental and contextual factors, such as the child's age at injury, stage of brain development, and functional maturation (Anderson, Catroppa, Morse, Haritou, & Rosenfeld, 2005b; Taylor & Alden, 1997); the key role of the family; and implications of life tasks specific to children (Yeates, Taylor, Drotar, Wade, et al., 1997).

Outcomes of Child TBI

To begin, in recognition of the very different acute consequences and later recovery trajectories associated with mild (that is, concussion, mild, and mild complicated) and more serious (moderate to severe) child TBI, we have separated our discussion of the literature relevant to each throughout the book.

Although some controversy remains, research has demonstrated that children with milder injuries are likely to recover well, with few residual problems. With increasing severity, recovery is less complete, and we know that those with severe injury are at risk for ongoing difficulties across a range of domains and that these difficulties may persist into adulthood (Hessen, Nestvold, & Anderson, 2007; Jaffe, Polissar, Fay, & Liao, 1995; Yeates, Swift, Taylor, Wade, et al., 2004).

Research findings, from a range of mostly discipline-specific research endeavors, describe an increased risk for a multitude of residual impairments following childhood TBI, both acute and long-term. Persisting neurological symptoms, motor dysfunction, communication difficulties, poor attention and information processing, reduced memory, executive dysfunction, and social and emotional disorders have been consistently reported for many children with serious TBI. In association with these impairments, functional outcomes are also affected, with solid evidence of low academic achievement, reduced vocational opportunities, poor adaptive skills, and lowered quality of life.

There remains a significant challenge for the direct application of these research-based findings, with clinical reports confirming that outcomes are highly variable and difficult to predict, leading to uncertainty with respect to prognosis and need for follow-up and treatment. For example, anecdotal clinical reports describe excellent recovery after severe TBI in some children. In contrast, emerging trends in the child concussion literature suggest that a subset of young people will experience delayed recovery, characterized by persistent and debilitating symptoms that affect participation in school and social activities and quality of life.

More precise information is critical to determine which children are at high risk for poorer outcomes and to effectively allocate management and treatment resources. To date, research has been only modestly successful in providing guidance with respect to which factors contribute most to recovery and positive outcomes. Much research on child TBI has focused on specific domains. For example, medical researchers may examine the impact of raised intracranial pressure or neurological signs on long-term outcomes, whereas others may look at specific biochemical markers, radiological results, or environmental factors. The fact that progress using such a narrow focus has been disappointing suggests that a more multi-dimensional model is required, in which researchers across disciplines come together with a more holistic view of the child, recognizing the likelihood that factors across multiple dimensions (e.g., injury, environment, developmental stage) interact to determine eventual outcomes. In support of this, *emerging research* suggests that the search for globally relevant markers of outcome may not be fruitful; rather, there may be differing markers for outcomes across specific domains. For example, injury factors may predict physical and cognitive recovery, whereas environmental factors may be more closely linked to behavior and socio-emotional outcomes.

Management, Treatment, and Intervention

A further challenge exists in the area of management and treatment. At present, evidence for effective treatment, at both acute and more long-term stages of recovery, is largely lacking across medical, pharmacological, cognitive, and behavioral domains (Anderson & Catroppa, 2006; Laatsch, Harrington, Hotz, Marcantuono, et al., 2007; Robinson, Kaizar, Catroppa, Godfrey, & Yeates, 2014; Ylvisaker, Adelson, Willandino Braga, Burnett, et al., 2005). As a result, health professionals have little direction with respect to which interventions may lead to better outcomes. Reflecting this problem, clinical practice guidelines, where established, vary dramatically across the world, and even within individual centers. Care pathways are disparate, and clinical decisions are typically based more on previous training and experience than on empirical grounds. Treatment research and clinical trials in this domain are costly and difficult, but they are critical to improving child outcomes.

A Bio-Psycho-Social Model of Child TBI

To understand child TBI and its outcomes, we suggest a developmentally driven "bio-psycho-social framework," integrating biological, neurobehavioral, and psychosocial/environmental dimensions, all of which contribute to the child's recovery from TBI. With respect to the *biological* dimension, initial brain insult due to TBI results in interruptions to cerebral circulation, changes in intracranial pressure, loss of tissue, and disruptions in neural networks. Such damage is associated with a characteristic set of *psychological* deficits in attention and memory, information processing, executive function, communication, and behavior and social skills, whether due to the direct effects of brain injury or as a "secondary consequence"—a consequence of adapting to the consequences of TBI (e.g., physical limitations, response to trauma). The quality of the child's *environment,* including family function, stress, and coping, as well as access to resources, has been identified as critical to long-term outcomes.

Of crucial importance is growing evidence for a *developmentally specific* response to injury, demonstrating that knowledge and theories regarding adult TBI cannot be simply translated to the child population. The relative vulnerability of the young brain to the impact of TBI and the increased behavioral consequences in terms of reduced skill and knowledge acquisition is a relatively new concept but is already supported by animal research, neuroimaging data, and behavioral findings. Over time, and in the context of ongoing *development,* cumulative problems may emerge. For instance, child TBI may lead to an interruption or deviation in normal developmental processes, both at a neuroanatomic level and at a neurobehavioral level. At the same time, the child's psychological function may become increasingly problematic, due to his or her failure to acquire appropriate cognitive, behavioral, and social skills. Such failure may hamper knowledge acquisition and consolidation while increasing social isolation and associated family stresses. The long-term consequences of these multiple and interacting factors may result in a picture of global dysfunction. This view is supported by an emerging literature that describes adult survivors of child TBI as experiencing academic failure, restricted vocational options, psychological adjustment difficulties, and poor quality of life (Anderson, Brown, Newitt, & Hoile, 2011; Cattelani, Lombardi, Brianti, & Mazzucchi, 1998; Di Battista, Godfrey, Soo, Catroppa, & Anderson, 2014; McKinlay, Dalrymple-Alford, Hoorwood, & Fergusson, 2002). The child's need to acquire new skills and knowledge and meet educational demands, in the context of increased risk of physical, cognitive, and behavioral impairment, generates unique challenges for rehabilitation and reintegration following TBI. Appropriate and timely intervention and follow-up, for both child and family—based on knowledge of the disorder, its symptomatology, and likely outcomes—may prevent such poor prognosis and enable the child and family to understand and successfully manage these problems.

As mentioned above, research on child TBI has often occurred in separate silos, with little integration across domains or disciplines. The scientific advances that have occurred within domains (e.g., genomics and proteomics of neural recovery, neuroimaging, neuropsychology) are unlikely to result in significant progress in the clinical management of children with TBI until such advances become the topic of collaborative research that cuts across levels and specialties. In the field of TBI, we can learn much from the study of other childhood disorders, such as childhood cancer, where international collaborative consortia have been in existence for many years and have led the way in developing and implementing evidence-based, life-saving treatment protocols that have reduced mortality rates from 70% (in the 1970s) to close to 10% (in the past decade).

Conclusions

The time seems ripe for an interdisciplinary and collaborative approach to pediatric TBI that promotes integrative and translational research efforts. We believe that this book, *New Frontiers in Pediatric Traumatic Brain Injury: An Evidence Base for Clinical Practice,* will help advance the state-of-the-art of research in the field and promote networking and collaboration among investigators. The chapters that constitute the book describe the state of the art in research across a variety of disciplines, all of which contribute to developing knowledge about pediatric TBI. This body of work makes it clear that the challenges and obstacles we face are similar regardless of discipline and that the solutions for progress will require a concerted investigation that cuts across disciplines and other artificial boundaries.

2

EPIDEMIOLOGY

Child traumatic brain injury (TBI) is the most frequent cause of interruption to normal development and results in significant impairments in many survivors. Not all children are at equal risk of sustaining a TBI, and predicting outcome is difficult. Long-term consequences depend on premorbid abilities, injury characteristics, environmental context, developmental stage, and access to rehabilitation, as well as factors yet to be identified.

Although injury severity is the best-established index of outcome, ongoing impairment has also been linked to premorbid learning and behavior problems, reduced access to intervention and support services post-injury, and environmental factors such as social disadvantage and family stress. Age and/or developmental level at the time of injury are further critical factors in the recovery from child TBI. Though some have argued that younger children recover better than adolescents and adults because their brains are more adaptable (or "plastic"), studies now show that the developing brain may be particularly vulnerable to early injury because of the potential for brain damage to disrupt critical stages of neural and cognitive maturation. The goal of this chapter is to provide an overview of the epidemiology of TBI sustained in childhood and to consider approaches to classification.

Accurate statistics regarding the incidence and prevalence of childhood TBI are difficult to obtain, with epidemiological studies varying widely in terms of injury definition, sources of data, data collection techniques, case descriptions, and ages of target populations. Population estimates of child TBI are usually based on deaths, hospitalizations, and emergency department presentations. Such estimates range between 250 and 799 per 100,000 per year (Crowe, Babl, Anderson, & Catroppa, 2009; Kraus, 1995; Langlois et al., 2006; Tate, McDonald, & Lulham, 1998). However, these figures fail to account for those children who present to community practitioners or who fail to seek any medical assistance. Highlighting the limitations of available data, the Christchurch birth cohort study has documented an average incidence of child TBI to be 1.10–2.36 per year, with an overall incidence of approximately 30% by age 25 years (McKinlay, Grace, Horwood, & Fergusson, 2008), as well as increased risk of multiple TBIs following an initial event. These authors also noted that many young people did not present to hospital but were more likely to visit their local doctor.

For children who do seek hospital care, approximately 80% will have mild injuries (Kraus, Fife, Cox, Ramstein, & Conroy, 1986; Lescohier & DiScala, 1993), half will have no loss of consciousness post-injury (Kraus et al., 1986), between 5 and 10 percent will experience temporary and/or permanent neuropsychological sequelae, and 5 to 10 percent will receive fatal injuries (Goldstein & Levin, 1987). One in every 30 newborn children will sustain a TBI before age 16 (Annegers, 1983). Examination of data relating specifically to children admitted to hospital with a severe TBI shows that the mortality rate is approximately one-third, with another third of child victims making a good recovery, and the last third exhibiting residual disability (Michaud, Rivara, Grady, & Reay, 1992). Such incidence levels establish TBI sustained in childhood as a significant community problem.

Over recent years, a variety of prevention initiatives have been developed with the aim of reducing the incidence of TBI, in particular severe TBI. For example, across the globe, seatbelt laws, helmet laws, and campaigns against drunk driving have reduced the overall death rate from motor vehicle accidents, as well as the incidence of severe TBI. Similar public health campaigns have targeted child abuse, substance abuse, and physical assault. More recently, with an increase in profile of sports concussions and mild head injuries, consideration has been given to the use of helmets and implementation of rules regarding return to school and play to minimize the opportunity for serial injuries. Though these various approaches are reported to have succeeded in reducing the overall number of incidents as well as the number of fatal and severe head injuries, few compelling data are available, and child TBI remains a significant community problem.

Emergency Department Presentation Rates and Cause of Injury

Our team (Crowe et al., 2009) recently conducted an audit of all cases presenting at the Royal Children's Hospital (RCH), Melbourne, Australia, over a 12-month period. To provide some context, the RCH is the only tertiary pediatric trauma center in the state of Victoria, which has a population of approximately 3 million. The RCH thus acts as the statewide catchment for significant child illnesses and injuries. It also serves as the primary health service for children living in metropolitan Melbourne. During the 12-month period covered by our audit, there were 54,233 presentations for all reasons. When searching the specified ICD-10 codes and criteria, we identified 1,115 cases of head injury, excluding concussions.

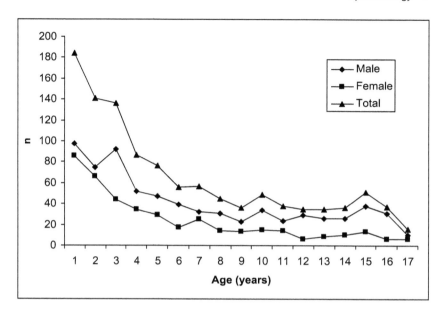

FIGURE 2.1

Source: From Crowe et al. (2009). Reprinted with permission of John Wiley & Sons.

There were 1,089 presentations to the ED; 26 (2.4%) of the children were admitted directly to the ICU and two died in the ICU from their injuries. In terms of injury severity, 89.1% were mild, 7.9% were moderate, and 3.0% were severe. Most children were from the Melbourne metropolitan area ($n = 1,006, 90.2\%$). The age- and gender-specific rates are displayed in Figure 2.1. Of note, in a more recent survey of children, restricted to 5–18 years of age, and presenting to the ED of the same hospital with a diagnosis of concussion (that is, reflecting presentations not covered in the Crowe et al., 2009 study), we captured over 500 children in a 12-month period, suggesting the rate of head injuries is likely much higher than previously reported.

Data regarding the cause of child TBI can provide important information about the mechanism of brain injuries, which vary across infancy and childhood (Koepsell, Rivara, Vavilala, Wang, et al., 2011). The most common causes of child TBI are transport-related accidents (passenger, bike rider, pedestrian), falls, and assaults, which together account for more than 50% of TBIs sustained under 10 years of age. Injuries due to sporting activities represent the single most common cause of injury in children over 10 years of age (Crowe et al., 2009; Langlois et al., 2006), as illustrated in Table 2.1. Infants and toddlers (0–4 years) are especially likely to sustain TBI via inflicted injuries secondary to child abuse (Adelson & Kochanek, 1998; Holloway, Bye, & Moran, 1994; Keenan & Bratton, 2006). Such injuries, sometimes called "shaken baby syndrome," demonstrate quite different features compared to other forms of TBI, which usually result from a single impact. Characteristically, they include multiple and diffuse pathology and often have serious secondary consequences, including hypoxia and hypotension. A study by Keenan

TABLE 2.1 External Causes of Head Injury by Age Group (%)

	0–2 yrs (n = 460)	3–5 yrs (n = 219)	6–8 yrs (n = 139)	9–11 yrs (n = 122)	12–14 yrs (n = 122)	15–16 yrs (n = 53)
Motor vehicle	3.5	9.1	7.9	10.7	10.7	13.2
Passenger	2.6	5.4	3.6	4.9	3.3	5.6
Bike	0.7	2.3	0.8	3.3	4.1	7.6
Pedestrian	0.2	1.4	3.6	2.5	3.3	—
Fall	74.4	62.1	46.8	36.1	22.1	11.4
Inflicted	0.7	1.4	3.6	2.5	9.0	20.8
Parent	0.7	—	—	—	—	1.7
Peer	—	1.4	3.6	2.5	9.0	19.1
Sports	7.2	21.0	38.1	45.9	54.2	47.3
Sport	0.9	9.1	18.7	37.7	51.7	47.3
Playground	6.3	11.9	19.4	8.2	2.5	—
Other	14.5	6.0	3.6	4.1	4.1	5.7

Source: From Crowe et al. (2009). Reprinted with permission of John Wiley & Sons.

and colleagues (Keenan, Runyan, Marshall, Nocera, et al., 2003) also reports that younger age, male gender, younger mother (< 21 years), and product of multiple birth were all risk factors for inflicted TBIs. Toddlers are also likely to be injured through falls, at home or during play (Crowe et al., 2009; Holloway et al., 1994). In older children, sports and recreational accidents, as well as pedestrian or bicycle collisions with motor vehicles, account for an increasing proportion of TBI. Adolescents are especially likely to be injured in motor vehicle collisions, with assaults also common in this age range.

With the recent increased interest in sports-related injuries, it is timely to look specifically at the causes of such injuries. In our audit of child presentations for TBI, we (Crowe et al., 2009) found that, over a 12-month period, there were 406 presentations to the RCH ED for TBI in school-aged children, with 33% related to sporting activities. Seventy percent of victims were male. Most injuries were classified as mild; 13% were classified as moderate or severe. Among a range of sports, Australian Rules Football was associated with more than 30% of all events attributable to a sport or recreation cause. Equestrian activities were the main cause of moderate TBI.

Mortality and Morbidity

Traumatic injuries account for the majority of deaths among children and adolescents, with 40% to 50% of these deaths associated with a TBI (Kraus, 1995). Overall, mortality rates are lower among children than among adolescents and adults, although infancy represents a particularly high-risk period. Estimates of mortality are around 4.5 per 100,000 per year for children 0–14 years of age, increasing to 24 per 100,000 for 15–19 year olds (Langlois et al., 2006). Not surprisingly, the mortality rate is highest among those with more severe injuries and virtually nil among those with mild injuries. In a comprehensive survey reported in 1995, Kraus found that, for severe injuries, the mortality rate was 12–62%, versus only 4% for moderate injuries and less than 1% for mild injuries (Kraus, 1995).

Survivors of child TBI frequently experience adverse consequences. In his review, Kraus (1995) found that between 75% and 95% of children with TBI displayed good recovery, about 10% showed a moderate disability, 1% to 3% showed a severe disability, and less than 1% remained in a persistent vegetative state. However, these figures were based on a global outcome scale, which did not comprehensively assess functional disabilities, neurobehavioral, and psychosocial impairments (Koelfen, Freund, Dinter, Schmidt, et al., 1997). More recent targeted studies report substantial and persisting morbidity in these domains which have a significant impact on survivors' quality of life and ability to participate fully in activities of daily life (e.g., school, leisure, sports).

Demographic Characteristics

Age: There is some evidence that patient fatality rates decrease as age increases. Michaud and colleagues (1992) report that, in their study of serious TBI, 14% of children injured over the age of 14 years died from their injury, whereas the fatality rate for children under 2 years was 50%. In addition, they found better recovery with increasing age. Death was most common in the under-2 age group, whereas the majority of children injured after the age of 14 were classified as showing good recovery. These data are consistent with the causes of injury across childhood, with inflicted injuries most common in infancy and more likely to have poor outcome, whereas sporting injuries are more common in older children and teenagers and are usually linked to milder insults and better recovery.

Crowe et al. (2009) demonstrate that, when examining hospital presentation for TBI, the highest proportion of presentations to pediatric trauma centers is for infants and toddlers, who accounted for 49% of all presentations over a 12-month period. The remainder of presentations spread fairly evenly across the age groups from 5 to 17 years.

Gender: As is commonly reported, boys and girls are not equally at risk of sustaining TBI, and the relative risk of injury for boys and girls changes across childhood. A comparison of gender ratios shows that, in children under age 2, the male-to-female ratio is approximately equal (Crowe et al., 2009). In contrast, school-aged males are more than twice as likely as age-matched females to suffer TBI (Kraus, 1995). Further, Kraus and colleagues (1986) note that the incidence of TBI increases in males through childhood and adolescence, with a relative decline for females during this time.

Girls are more likely to sustain a TBI as a result of a fall or as a passenger in a car (Berney, Favier, & Froidevaux, 1994). Boys tend to sustain more severe trauma, with the mortality rate for male over female children estimated to be around 4:1

(Annegers, 1983). Lehr (1990) suggests that such gender differences, which have been consistently identified, may reflect higher levels of activity and exploratory behavior in boys.

Timing and location of injury: Epidemiological research demonstrates that child TBI occurs most frequently during the warmer months, with less than 10% of children sustaining their injuries during winter, mostly due to winter sports. Injuries are also most common on weekends, on holidays, and in the late afternoon/ early evening, when children are more likely to be involved in leisure activities. In fact, Crowe et al. (2009) report that, although school holidays constitute around 12% of the year, TBIs during this period accounted for more than 25% of annual presentations. Further, the majority of injuries occur in the home (57.1%), followed by a public place, including roads (13.1%). A small number of children are injured at schools (9.0%), sporting venues (7.7%), and playgrounds (5.7%). This pattern of findings has recently been replicated by Andersson, Sejdhage, & Wage (2012).

Child and family factors: It has been argued that many TBIs result from reckless behaviors in poorly supervised environments (Chadwick, Rutter, Brown, Shaffer, & Traub, 1981; Dalby & Obrzut, 1991). Further, it is often stated that TBI is more common in families in which parents are socially disadvantaged, unemployed, or emotionally disturbed (Anderson, Morse, Klugg, Catroppa, et al., 1997; Brown, Chadwick, Shaffer, Rutter, & Traub, 1981; Parslow, Morris, Tasker, Forsyth, & Hawley, 2005; Rivara, Jaffe, Fay, et al., 1993; Taylor, Drotar, Wade, Yeates, et al., 1995), in families in which parental neglect and poor supervision are evident (Moyes, 1980), and in children with pre-existing learning and behavioral deficits (Asarnow, Satz, Light, Zaucha, et al., 1995; Brown et al., 1981; Ponsford, Willmott, Rothwell, Cameron, et al., 1999). Recent research suggests that the relevance of these psychosocial factors may also change with age. For example, parent mental health and family function have been found to be associated with TBI in younger children. Specifically, parents with high stress (single parents, those with financial difficulties, and those with mental health diagnoses) are over-represented in samples of infants and toddlers with TBI. In contrast, for older children, it appears that the child's own behaviors (e.g., hyperactivity, inattention) may be more likely to increase the risk of TBI. In the US, studies have reported higher rates of hospitalization and death following motor vehicle accidents for black children (Langlois et al., 2006), whereas in the UK studies have linked social disadvantage to more severe child TBI (Parslow et al., 2005).

Community Costs of Child TBI

The costs to the community from TBI are significant. In the US, direct medical costs and indirect costs, such as lost productivity of TBI survivors, totaled an estimated $76.5 billion in 2000 (Finkelstein, Corso, Miller, & Associates, 2006) of TBI at any age. Child TBI specific figures within the UK indicate the lifetime costs associated with a serious child TBI total £4.9 million per child, with the greater proportion of this amount being accounted for by missed employment (£1.7 million), government benefits (£1.1 million), and direct social costs (£1.1 million).

In Australia, based on recent figures, the total community cost of TBI has been estimated at $9 billion per year, with costs divided among the individual/family (64.9%), the state (19.1%), and the federal government (11.1%). Following adult TBI, the lifetime cost per individual is reported to be $5 million for severe injury and $3.7 million for moderate injury (Access Economics, 2009). Though no such estimates are available for children, it is reasonable to assume that, for the preschool child, who has 60 or more years to live, the associated costs are likely far greater, especially if functional problems (e.g., physical, cognitive, social) are not recognized and treated early. In addition to the significant health costs associated with pediatric TBI (e.g., acute medical care, ongoing rehabilitation, medication), many children will also require mental health interventions across the life span, as well as substantial educational and vocational assistance. Long-term costs may include loss of earnings and carer support. Family costs, in terms of increased stress and burden, loss of earning, and mental health problems, are also common.

3

MECHANISMS AND PATHOPHYSIOLOGY

Terminology

The scientific literature on head injuries is filled with a confusing array of overlapping terms and constructs, among them *concussion, minor head injury, mild complicated head injury, head injury,* and *traumatic brain injury*. All of these terms refer to trauma caused by an external mechanical force. Each has a slightly different meaning and history, partially reflecting whether underlying cerebral injury is presumed. The term *concussion* (or *commotio cerebri*) has been used for centuries to imply a transient loss or alteration of consciousness without associated structural damage. In recent years, "concussion" has come to be used most frequently in reference to sports-related head trauma. *Minor head injury* is the broadest of the terms and includes not only craniocerebral trauma but extracranial injury as well. *Mild complicated head injury* is a more recent addition, and it generally refers to concussion or mild head injury in which unexpected cerebral pathology is detected or in which recovery is more protracted than expected. *Head injury* and *traumatic brain injury* are often used interchangeably, though technically only *TBI* implies the presence of cerebral injury. Throughout the following discussion, we primarily use the term *TBI*, as our focus is on individuals who have sustained trauma to the brain.

Penetrating and Closed-Head Injuries

Traumatic brain injuries can be classified into *penetrating* and *closed injuries*. The hallmark of *penetrating injuries*, as the term suggests, is penetration of the skull by some form of missile—usually a bullet, rock, or knife. This type of injury accounts for approximately 10% of all instances of child TBI. In penetrating head injury, cerebral pathology tends to be localized around the path of the missile.

Additionally, damage may result from penetrating skull fragments or shattered fragments from the missile itself. Secondary damage may occur due to cerebral infection (from the alien object entering the brain), swelling, bleeding, and raised intracranial pressure. Though loss of consciousness is relatively uncommon following penetrating head injury, neurologic deficits and post-traumatic epilepsy are frequently observed, and these are much more prevalent following penetrating head injury than closed-head injury.

Neurobehavioral sequelae from penetrating head injury tend to reflect the focal nature of the lesion sustained. Children usually exhibit quite specific deficits consistent with the localization of the lesion, with other skills relatively intact. Though these specific impairments are likely to persist, there is an opportunity to use intact abilities to develop compensatory strategies, or "alternate routes" for coping with cognitive demands.

Closed-head injury refers specifically to head injuries that do not involve penetration of the skull and dural layer (themselves called *penetrating/perforating* or *open-head injuries*). Closed-head injury accounts for the majority of instances of child TBI. In closed-head injury, the skull is not penetrated, but the brain is shaken around within the skull cavity, resulting in multiple injury sites, as well as diffuse axonal damage (See figure 3.1). The most common cause of such injuries is motor vehicle accidents, which are associated with high-velocity deceleration forces. A closed-head injury, however, can result from either direct or indirect impact via acceleration-deceleration injury (Andriessen, Jacobs, & Vos, 2010; Feng, Abney, Okamoto, Pless, et al., 2010; Gaetz, 2004). A blow to the head results in a direct head injury, whereas indirect injuries may result from jarring of the brain against the skull or rotational acceleration-deceleration forces resulting in shearing injuries. *Coup-contrecoup* injuries result from a combination of direct and indirect forces, where a blow to one side of the skull results in the brain being jarred inside the skull, hitting the side opposite the blow (Andriessen et al., 2010; Barkhoudarian, Hovda, & Giza, 2011).

Rotational acceleration usually occurs with the presence of rotation about the center of gravity of the brain, with no movement to the center of gravity itself. It usually involves the corpus callosum and the brain stem, affecting consciousness of an individual. Because rotational acceleration produces high surface strain and high levels of strain deep within the brain itself, it is a substantially critical and injurious mechanism. Conversely, translational acceleration happens when the center of gravity of the brain moves in a straight line, producing various focal injuries, such as *contrecoup* contusion and intracerebral and subdural hematomas. Angular acceleration, on the other hand, involving both translational and rotational movements, represents the most injurious brain injury mechanism, resulting in almost every known type of head injury (Gennarelli & Thibault, 1982; Guskiewicz & Mihalik, 2011; Yoganandran, Baisden, Maiman, Gennarelli, et al., 2010).

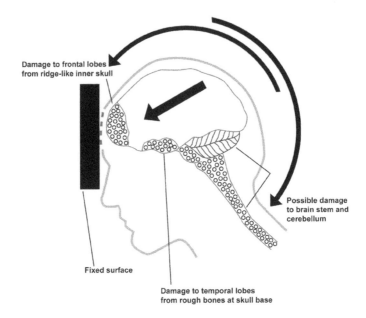

Damage to frontal lobes from ridge-like inner skull

Fixed surface

Possible damage to brain stem and cerebellum

Damage to temporal lobes from rough bones at skull base

Acceleration/Deceleration Injury

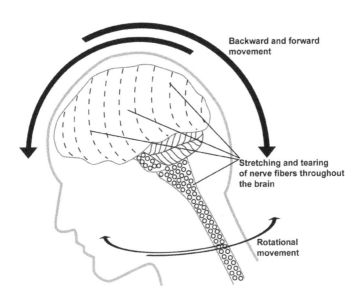

Backward and forward movement

Stretching and tearing of nerve fibers throughout the brain

Rotational movement

Whiplash Injury

FIGURE 3.1 Rotational Acceleration-Deceleration Causing Shearing Injury to Nerve Fibers

Source: Reprinted with permission of The Brain Center for Neurological Rehabilitation, Colorado.

Pathophysiology

The pathophysiology of TBI results from compression and deformation of the skull and begins at the time of impact but continues over a period of days, weeks, or even longer. Indeed, recent research indicates that the brain damage resulting from TBI involves more complex, prolonged, and interwoven processes than was previously recognized (Farkas & Povlishock, 2007; Giza & Hovda, 2001; Povlishock & Katz, 2005). The consequences of child TBI may be different from those observed in adults, as the immature brain responds differently to trauma than the mature brain (Giza, Mink, & Madikians, 2007). Research has found that children are more likely to suffer from post-traumatic brain swelling, hypoxic–ischemic insult, and diffuse, rather than focal, injuries, but less likely to present with intracranial hematomas. Compared to adults, children have a greater head-to-body ratio, less myelination, and greater relative proportion of water content and cerebral blood volume. Once children reach adolescence, TBI-related pathology begins to more closely resemble that seen in adults.

The typical pathophysiology of TBI may be classified based on the relationship to the initial insult (see Table 3.1). *Primary impact injuries* occur as a direct result of the application of force to the brain; they include skull fractures,

TABLE 3.1 Neuropathology of TBI

Type of Insult	*Neuropathology*
Primary	Skull fracture
	Intracranial contusions and laceration
	Diffuse axonal injury
Secondary	Brain swelling
	Cerebral edema
	Elevated intracranial pressure
	Hypoxia-ischemia
	Mass lesions (hematoma)
Neurochemical	Excessive production of free radicals
	Excessive release of excitatory neurotransmitters
	Alterations in glucose metabolism
	Decreased cerebral blood flow
Late/delayed	White matter degeneration and cerebral atrophy
	Post-traumatic hydrocephalus
	Post-traumatic seizures

Source: Adapted from Yeates (2010).

contusions and lacerations, and diffuse axonal damage. Such injuries are generally permanent and show little response to early treatment. *Secondary injuries* occur as a consequence of the primary injury. Raised intracranial pressure and brain swelling are two major secondary complications that are particularly common in children (Kochanek, 2006), while hypoxia and infection, as well as metabolic changes including hypothermia, electrolyte imbalance, and respiratory difficulties, may also occur (Begali, 1992; North, 1984; Pang, 1985). Secondary injuries have been found to be predictive of poor outcome (Quattrocchi, Prasad, Willits, & Wagner, 1991), but are also more responsive to appropriate and timely medical interventions.

Features of Primary Injury

Skull fractures are relatively common features of traumatic brain injury. Whereas linear fractures tend to be relatively benign, depressed, compound, and comminuted fractures are more serious and are often associated with other primary and secondary problems (e.g., lacerations, secondary bleeds, raised intracranial pressure). *Cerebral contusions* refer to bruising of the brain due to damage to internal tissue and blood vessels, resulting in bleeding and swelling. Focal contusions are especially likely to occur in the frontal and temporal cortex, because of its proximity to the bony prominences in the anterior and middle fossa of the skull (Bigler, 2007), and neuroimaging consistently reveals an anterior-posterior gradient in the focal lesions associated with TBI. Focal lesions are generally larger, and occur more frequently in, frontal and anterior temporal regions than in posterior temporal, parietal, or occipital regions (Wilde, Hunter, Newsome, Scheibel, et al., 2005). *Cerebral laceration* involves tearing of brain tissue as a result of a foreign object or pushed-in bone fragment from a skull fracture (Hardman & Manoukian, 2002). Lacerations tend to occur with other brain injuries—in particular, skull fractures.

Diffuse axonal injury (DAI) is a common characteristic in TBI (Cloots, van Dommelen, Nyberg, Lleiven, & Geers, 2011; Kelly & Rosenberg, 1997; Skandsen, Kvistad, Solheim, Strand, et al., 2010; Xu, Rasmussen, Lagopoulos, & Haberg, 2007). It is due to angular or rotational forces imparted on the brain during a traumatic injury. These forces result in twisting and shearing of brain tissue, leading to tearing or breaking of delicate axons (see Figure 3.2). DAI is often widespread, causing microscopic damage, and is associated with significant long-term functional disabilities (Levin, Wilde, Troyanskaya, Petersen, et al., 2010; Matsukawa, Shinoda, Fujii, Takahashi, et al., 2011; Skandsen et al., 2010; Wilde, Chu, Bigler, Hunter, et al., 2006; Xu et al., 2007). However, DAI appears to be most common at the boundaries between gray and white matter, and such injury tends to occur most often around the basal ganglia, periventricular regions, superior cerebellar peduncles, fornices, corpus callosum, and fiber tracts of the brain stem.

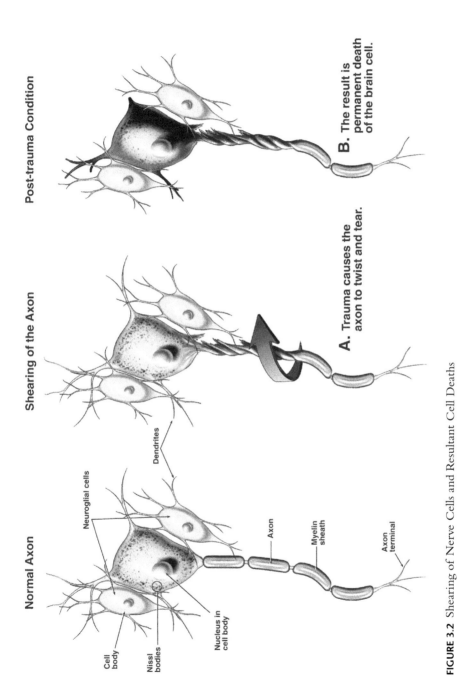

Normal Axon

Neuroglial cells

Dendrites

Cell body

Nissl bodies

Nucleus in cell body

Axon

Myelin sheath

Axon terminal

Shearing of the Axon

A. Trauma causes the axon to twist and tear.

Post-trauma Condition

B. The result is permanent death of the brain cell.

FIGURE 3.2 Shearing of Nerve Cells and Resultant Cell Deaths

Secondary Injuries

Secondary brain injuries can be defined as cell injury that is not present immediately after the primary brain injury / primary impact. These may develop over a period of hours or days following the initial traumatic injury. Further destruction of brain tissue most commonly occurs as a result of changes at the cellular or vascular level in the brain (Aronowski & Zhao, 2011; Jeremitski, Omert, Dunham, Wilberger, & Rodriguez, 2005). Of note, secondary brain damage is potentially preventable and treatable given appropriate acute management.

Though less common in children than adults, mass effects, often related to vascular interruptions, lead to increased cerebral volume and raised intracranial pressure. If not treated quickly, usually via surgical evacuation, these secondary complications may cause cerebral herniation and ultimately death. The major types of hematoma are epidural, subdural, and intracerebral, with these labels defining the site of the blood collection. Epidural and subdural hematoma are situated within the meningeal coverings of the brain. *Epidural hematomas* refer to bleeds above the dura, just below the surface of the skull, and not directly involving brain tissue. They are usually related to a skull fracture, where vessels in the meninges have been damaged. *Subdural hematomas* present as a collection between the dura and the arachnoid mater, resulting from injury to the blood vessels in the cortex or injury to the venous sinuses (Figure 3.3). These are more common and serious than epidural collections, mostly occurring as a consequence of massive cortical disruption and lacerations to blood vessels within the brain, where the underlying damaged brain may undergo rapid edema formation leading to mass effect, requiring surgical evacuation. *Intracerebral hematomas* occur within the brain parenchyma and often follow the same spatial distribution as contusions. They may result from shear injuries to brain tissue. When these complications are treated promptly,

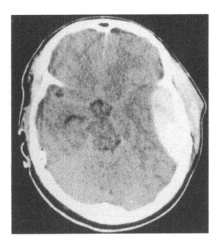 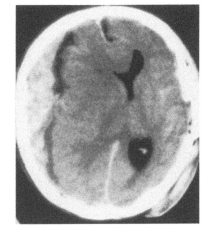

FIGURE 3.3 (a) Epidural Hematoma (b) Subdural Hematoma

outcome is good (Michaud et al., 1992). If left untreated, increasing blood mass may cause cerebral shift and herniation.

Cerebral edema, or brain swelling, refers to an increase in fluid volume within the skull, and it can be fatal when it causes raised intracranial pressure, preventing blood from entering the brain. Edema is thought to result from disruption of normal relationships between blood, brain tissue, and cerebrospinal fluid, which results in decreased cerebral blood flow, increased cerebral blood volume, and increased intracranial pressure, due to a failure of the autoregulatory mechanism of cerebral blood flow, hypoxia, hypercapnea, or obstruction to cerebral circulation. Together these factors can lead to ischemic and hypoxic injury, as well as brain herniation and death (Bruce, 1995; Pang, 1985). Any increase in the content of the brain (that is, brain, cerebrospinal fluid, cerebral blood volume, extracellular fluid) will cause increased intracranial pressure. In the case of TBI, the presence of brain swelling or hematoma is the primary cause of raised intracranial pressure. Intracranial pressure is routinely monitored following TBI, and surgical treatment may be required to reduce pressure in some patients.

Neurochemical and Neurometabolic Mechanisms

Recent research has suggested that further secondary damage may be due to neurochemical processes, mediated by a cascade of biochemical and metabolic reactions following a TBI (Farkas & Povlishock, 2007; Novack, Dillon, & Jackson, 1996; Prins, Giza, & Hovda, 2010). TBI can result in a variety of neurochemical events, including the production of free radicals and excitatory amino acids and the disruption of normal calcium homeostasis, as well as changes in glucose metabolism and cerebral blood flow (Giza & Hovda, 2001). These events act in concert to exacerbate the hypoxic-ischemic insult that commonly occurs following TBI (Figure 3.4). Animal research suggests that pharmacological interventions may be successful in reducing brain injury due to such mechanisms (Novack et al., 1996), although the results of human trials have so far been disappointing.

Late Effects

Though relatively uncommon following closed-head injury, a number of delayed medical complications may also develop in the sub-acute stages post-injury. Communicating hydrocephalus may occur when there is an obstruction of the flow of cerebrospinal fluid, often due to vascular disruption (McLean, Kaitz, Kennan, Dabney, et al., 1995). Cerebral infections may arise in association with skull fractures. These infections usually take the form of meningitis or cerebral abscess. Each of these complications may be detected on the basis of increased intracranial pressure and associated late deterioration in function.

Following closed-head injury, patients also have increased risk of epilepsy. Early seizures, defined as occurring within the first week after TBI, occur in many

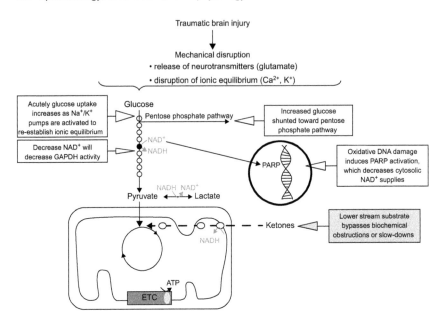

FIGURE 3.4 Diagram of the Biochemical Changes After TBI

Source: From Prins et al. (2010). Reprinted with permission of Cambridge University Press.

children and can involve focal status epilepticus (Statler, 2006). Very young children seem especially vulnerable to such seizures. The occurrence of seizures soon after injury does not necessarily place children at risk for later epilepsy, which occurs in about 10–20% of children with severe TBI. Post-traumatic epilepsy is more common in children with penetrating injuries, inflicted injuries, or depressed skull fracture, all of which are indicative of focal pathology (Jennett & Bond, 1975; Pang, 1985; Raimondi & Hirschauer, 1984). Most post-traumatic seizures occur within two years of injury and have been linked to poor outcome (Anderson, Brown, Newitt, & Hoile, 2009).

Neuroimaging studies demonstrate that severe TBI in particular can be associated with a gradual and prolonged process of white-matter degeneration and cortical thinning, with associated cerebral atrophy and ventricular enlargement. Ventricular dilatation can also occur due to disruption of the circulation of cerebrospinal fluid (Ghosh, Wilde, Hunter, Bigler, et al., 2009; Merkley, Bigler, Wilde, McCauley, et al., 2008).

Conclusions

There has been relatively little progress over recent decades with respect to understanding the patterns and prevalence of child TBI. Further, methods for diagnosing injury, determining severity, managing potentially preventable secondary consequences, and predicting outcomes remain inaccurate.

4

ASSESSING ACUTE ASPECTS
OF CHILD TBI

The complex pathophysiology of pediatric TBI necessitates in-depth assessment of the brain injury itself, as well as its medical and functional consequences. Children with brain injury come under the responsibility of a number of clinical departments, each with their own focus and diagnostic and observational tools.

Paramedical, Acute, and Intensive Care Medical Assessment

Most emergency departments routinely evaluate severity using a number of specific measures, leading to a severity grading ranging from mild to severe.

Assessing level of consciousness. Loss of consciousness, or coma, is defined as a state in which there is no opening of the eyes (even in response to pain), no recognizable verbal response, and an inability to obey commands (Miller, 1991). It usually results from direct damage or dysfunction to the brain stem or from deafferentation through diffuse axonal injury. The Glasgow Coma Scale (Teasdale & Jennett, 1974) is a commonly employed measure to indicate level of consciousness in TBI patients. Assessment of duration of loss of consciousness and post-traumatic amnesia also provide information relevant to injury severity. In addition to assessing consciousness, the health care team investigates cerebral pathology, usually via CT scan initially, and then MRI scanning where further complications are suspected (this will be addressed in Chapter 5). These techniques provide the neurosurgical team with information regarding the need for surgical intervention—for example, where a bleed is present, causing mass effect and brain shift, or where raised intracranial pressure is evident, requiring drainage. Neurological examination is also performed to identify any neurological anomalies, which may help in localising cerebral damage.

The Glasgow Coma Scale. In the case of accidental injuries, assessment and diagnosis of TBI is generally initiated at the scene of the accident by emergency first responders, who perform preliminary determination of conscious state and neurological status. Most commonly, this will involve initial assessment of consciousness level using the modified Glasgow Coma Scale, originally developed by Teasdale and Jennett (1974). The greatest advantage of the GCS, and its adapted versions, is its wide usage, which provides benchmarks for injury severity. The GCS consists of a 15-point system, including assessment of eye opening, motor response, and verbal response. The best eye response is graded on four points (1—no eye opening; 2—eye opening in response to pain; 3—eye opening to speech; 4—eyes open spontaneously), the best verbal response is graded on five points (1—no verbal response; 2—incomprehensible sounds; 3—inappropriate speech; 4—confused; 5—oriented), and the best motor response is graded on a six-point scale (1—no motor response; 2—extension to pain (decerebrate response); 3—abnormal flexion to pain (decorticate response); 4—flexion/withdrawal to pain; 5—localization to pain; 6—obeys commands; see Table 4.1). The sub-scale values are considered separately, and they are also summed for an overall indication of severity level based on the following scores: mild TBI (GCS = 13–15), moderate (GCS = 8–12), and severe (GCS = 3–7).

TABLE 4.1 Comparison of Glasgow Coma Scale and Pediatric Coma Scale

Glasgow Coma Scale		Pediatric Coma Scale		Age-related best response
Eyes open				
Spontaneously	4	As for adults		As for adults
To speech	3			
To pain	2			
None	1			
Best motor response				
Obeys commands	6			
Localizes pain	5	As for adults		> 2 years
Withdraws	4			6 months–2 years
Flexion to pain	3			≤ 6 months
Extension to pain	2			
None	1			
Best verbal response				
Orientated	5	Orientated	5	> 5 years
Confused	4	Words	4	1–5 years
Words	3	Vocal sounds	3	26–52 weeks
Sounds	2	Cries	2	0–26 weeks
None	1	None	1	

Source: Adapted from Ruijs et al (1992).

Although the GCS remains the gold standard both in initial assessment of TBI and for classification of injury severity, it has come under criticism for a variety of reasons. First, there are subjective assessment aspects of the scale, and its reliability therefore depends on the experience of the rater (Rowley & Fielding, 1991). Second, it is unclear what acute injury time point yields the most predictive value of the GCS because of rapid changes incurred by brain injury. A GCS score at the scene of the accident may deteriorate or improve on reassessment in the emergency room as a result of intracranial injury or rapid recovery of consciousness. Third, the validity of these scores is compromised in cases of tracheal intubation and can be affected by medication administered acutely (e.g., sedation), which can nullify the use of the verbal response scale. Fourth, the GCS was derived to focus specifically on alterations in conscious state in the context of more severe injuries and thus will be less sensitive to the degree of severity in milder TBI, in which loss of consciousness is, by definition, brief. Further, evaluation of infants and preschool children is especially problematic because of the limitations associated with assessing verbal response in preverbal children and because some verbal and motor responses require a level of development not achieved until late childhood. To counter this, a pediatric version of the GCS has been developed (Pediatric GCS; Reilly, Simpson, Sprod, & Thomas, 1988) with special considerations for infants/children under the age of 5 for the verbal response scale (1—no response; 2—moans/incomprehensible words or nonspecific sounds; 3—cries/inappropriate words; 4—irritable cries/confused; 5—coos and babbles/oriented, appropriate speech; see Table 4.1). Given the lack of reliability of verbal responses in children, behavioral changes are of particular importance, and parents as well as emergency medical staff should pay special attention to personality, mood changes, and excessive crying.

Vital and neurological signs. Assessment of TBI on the scene and in the emergency room also involves documentation of history of the accident (if witnessed), any initial physical signs and symptoms through secondary survey, and observations that may suggest altered consciousness, brain injury, or other complications. Airway, breathing, and circulation are part of any standard emergency assessment, as are monitoring of vital signs (e.g., blood pressure, heart rate, temperature, respiration rate). Neurological and medical signs may include seizures, nausea and vomiting, sensory alterations (ringing in the ears, pain, tingling, or numbness), headache, visual problems such as diplopia (double vision), speech problems (aphasia, slurred or slowed speech), and vertigo/dizziness or light-headedness, as well as motor coordination and balance problems. Pupil reactivity and eye size also provide indications of underlying brain injury. Few signs of specific cognitive alteration are immediately notable; however, children and adolescents who suffer TBI may have acute memory loss (e.g., amnesia for the event), difficulty concentrating, and general disorientation and confusion. These cognitive signs are usually accompanied by acute behavioral changes, including emotional lability, irritability, anxiety, disinhibition, and impulsivity.

Post-Traumatic Amnesia and Ongoing Medical Assessment

Emergency room (ER) assessment of pediatric TBI follows on from information initially gathered at the scene leading to more in-depth observation, complete neurological and clinical evaluation, and follow-up as required by injury severity. Reassessment of conscious state is essential upon emergency-room presentation, because consciousness may fluctuate in association with underlying brain injury. Though some mild injuries may be accompanied by an improvement in GCS score between initial paramedical assessment and ER presentation as acute confusion clears, more severe injuries may inversely be accompanied by dramatic drops in GCS as underlying parenchymal injury ("neuroworsening") sets in.

Monitoring of post-traumatic amnesia (PTA; also called "post-traumatic con-fusional state") is considered a good indicator of the evolution of the injury. PTA refers to a period of confusion and disorientation, as well as loss of memories for events immediately preceding the injury (retrograde amnesia) and/or problems remembering events following the injury (anterograde amnesia). PTA may occur regardless of loss of consciousness or may be characteristic of the post-coma period of recovery. In addition to GCS scores, length of PTA is used as an indicator of injury severity (see Table 4.2), and some studies suggest that it is a better prog-nostic measure than the GCS (e.g., Brooks, Aughton, Bond, Jones, & Rizvi, 1980; Shores, 1989). Tools assessing PTA require serial administration in the days follow-ing the injury, until the child reaches criterion. The Westmead PTA Scale (Shores, Marosszeky, Sandanam, & Batchelor, 1986) is a commonly used measure, consisting of seven orientation questions and five memory items. PTA is said to have resolved when a patient achieves a perfect score on the scale for three consecutive days, and the first of those days is then identified as the day PTA ended. Because of its reliance on cognitive and verbal function, assessment of PTA in infants and young children is problematic. As a result, the Westmead Scale is considered appropriate only for children over the age of 8 years. For younger children, a modification of the Westmead PTA scale has been proposed and validated in children 4–5 years (Rocca, Wallen, & Batchelor, 2008). Alternatively, the Children's Orientation and Amnesia Test (Ewing-Cobbs, Levin, Fletcher, Miner, & Eisenberg, 1990), which consists of 16 items that assess general orientation, temporal orientation, and memory in children and was normed in 146 children between the ages of 3 and 15 years (Table 4.3), may

TABLE 4.2 Indices of Injury Severity

	Mild TBI	Moderate TBI	Severe TBI
Glasgow Coma Score	13–15	9–12	13–15
Loss of consciousness	< 30 mins	30 mins – 24 hrs	> 24 hrs
Post-traumatic amnesia	0–1 day	1–7 days	> 7 days

Source: Adapted from DeCuypere & Klimo (2012).

TABLE 4.3 The Children's Orientation and Amnesia Test (COAT)

General Orientation
1. What is your name (first, last)?
2. How old are you? When is your birthday (month, year)?
3. Where do you live (city, state)?
4. What is your father's name? What is your mother's name?
5. What school do you go to? What grade are you in?
6. Where are you now?
7. Is it daytime or nighttime?

Temporal Orientation
8. What time is it now?
9. What day of the week is it?
10. What day of the month is it?
11. What is the month?
12. What is the year?

Memory
13. Say these numbers after me in the same order.
    (strings of numbers of increasing length are presented to the child for recall)
14. How many fingers am I holding up?
15. Who is on *Sesame Street* (or substitute other TV show)?
16. What is my name?

Source: Adapted from Ewing Cobbs et al. (1990).

be used. Evaluation of PTA in children below the age of 3 is not currently possible based on any standardized scale.

As with the GCS, PTA measures are not particularly sensitive in the context of mild TBI, in which PTA may be brief and the child is not hospitalized for long enough to gain a reliable assessment.

Ongoing documentation of neurological, cognitive, and behavioral signs dictates management decisions. Assessment for some children may conclude with a short stay (commonly four to eight hours) in the emergency room or Short Stay Unit (where available) to monitor symptoms. Those with suspected brain injury and other complications (e.g., raised intracranial pressure, seizures) will be referred for neuroimaging assessment and to the intensive care unit for assessment of critical signs and symptoms (intracranial pressure, oxygen saturation, carbon dioxide, etc.), as well as for treatment.

A particular consideration in the acute medical assessment of child TBI is sensitivity to the presence of "inflicted" TBI, also referred to as non-accidental TBI and formerly "shaken baby syndrome." Though there is no pathognomonic sign for non-accidental TBI, initial assessment can reveal some indications that raise suspicion of abuse, though caution and adequate documentation must be exercised because of the social and legal implications of such a diagnosis. History taking is a particularly important aspect of non-accidental injury assessment, as studies show that lack of consistency in medical history may alert physicians to undeclared information. Some physical evidence is more likely to be associated with inflicted TBI, such as retinal hemorrhage, which is rarely seen after accidental TBI (Duhaime et al., 1987). In the absence of history of major trauma, skeletal surveys revealing multiple fractures may also raise suspicion of physical abuse (for detailed reviews on assessment characteristics of non-accidental brain injury, see Barnes, 2011; Maguire et al., 2009; Runyan, 2008; Runyan, Berger, & Barr, 2008).

A number of other scales exist for initial or acute assessment of brain injury severity and are frequently paired with the Glasgow Coma Scale.

The Rancho Los Amigos Scale Levels of Cognitive Functioning (LOCF). The LOCF (Hagen, 1998) is more detailed than the GCS and designed to measure cognitive and behavioral status as a patient emerges from coma. The scale includes eight levels of response and awareness to light, sound, touch, and commands. Because return to conscious state often occurs after emergency assessment, nurses (and occupational, speech, or physical therapists) frequently administer this scale as a basis for planning targeted assessments or interventions. The original scale was designed for children above the age of 14, but child versions exist for infants and for 2–5-year-olds.

The Disability Rating Scale (DRS). The DRS (Rappaport & Hall, 1982) includes three subscales that are similar to the GCS (eye opening, communication ability, and motor response), but it is designed to measure general functional changes over the course of recovery and therefore includes additional items relating to feeding, toileting, and grooming. Two additional subscales are included: level of functioning (physical, mental, emotional, or social function) and employability. As such, the DRS is usually used in rehabilitation settings. A maximum score of 29 indicates extreme vegetative state, whereas a score of zero indicates complete absence of disability. The DRS's advantage over other scales is its ability to track functional status from an acute time point (e.g., coma) to a chronic time point (e.g., community reintegration). The DRS is appropriate for use in adolescents and adults with moderate and severe TBI, but it has not been validated in younger children.

The Abbreviated Injury Scale (AIS). The AIS is an anatomical injury scoring system that uses a scale of 1 to 6 to rank injury severity (1—minor; 2—moderate; 3—serious; 4—severe; 5—critical; 6—unsurvivable). Though it is not a direct evaluation of brain injury per se, clinicians and researchers may encounter scores on the AIS (Copes, Sacco, Champion, & Bain, 1989) in relation to head injury and polytrauma. Of note, the scale is not a comprehensive assessment of injury and is not linear (e.g., the difference between levels 1 and 2 is not the same as between levels 5 and 6). It is suitable for indicating "threat to life" associated with an injury.

Sidelines Assessment: Tools for Acute Assessment of Sports Concussion

Mild TBI, or concussion, is common in a number of contact sports played by children and adolescents, especially hockey, soccer, and football. Sideline assessment of sports-related head injuries often follows a distinct path because of the need to quickly determine the severity of the blow and evaluate the need for further medical assessment, rest, or return-to-play. The Sport Concussion Assessment Tool (SCAT2; McCrory, Meeuwisse, Johnston, Dvorak, et al., 2009), as well as the Standardized Assessment of Concussion (SAC; McCrea, 2001a, 2001b; McCrea, Kelly, & Randolph, 2000; McCrea et al., 1998; McCrea, Kelly, Kluge, Ackley, & Randolph, 1997) and ImPACT sideline evaluation card (Bruce, Echemendia, Meeuwisse, Comper, & Sisco, 2014; Lovell & Collins, 1998; Lovell, Collins, Iverson, Field, et al., 2003; Lovell, Collins, Podell, Powell, & Maroon, 2000; McKay, Brooks, Mrazik, Jubinville, & Emery, 2014), are commonly used for immediate evaluation of sports concussion.

Over recent years, in recognition of the high numbers of children and youth sustaining concussive injuries, some of these measures have been modified for use with young people. The Child-SCAT, or the Sports Concussion Tool for Children age 5–12 years, has recently been developed but requires thorough standardization (Figure 4.1). The Child-SCAT includes the GCS, a child version of the Maddocks questions (Where are we now? Is it before or after lunch? What is your teacher's name? What did you have last lesson/class?), evaluation of post-concussive symptoms (parent and child report), a brief cognitive screen drawn from the SAC (McCrea, 2001a, 2001b: orientation, immediate memory, concentration), and examination of neck, balance, and overall coordination.

Advances in Acute Medical Assessment: Biomarkers

Though not part of standard clinical assessment, research in neuroproteomics suggests there are a number of acutely measurable brain biomarkers, which may be useful in predicting medical and functional outcome after child TBI. The mechanical forces sustained through TBI unleash a cascade of molecular events in the brain, including release of neurotransmitters and inflammatory processes resulting in cell death. These pathophysiological changes also affect the blood-brain barrier, causing cerebral edema and in some cases intracranial hypertension, thus resulting in secondary injury to the brain. Though biomarker research has not yet translated into clinical practice, identification of serum protein biomarkers released across the blood-brain barrier during the acute injury process shows promise in contributing to TBI assessment, diagnosis, and prediction of outcome. Immunoassay techniques are available to measure serum biomarkers as they are released and fluctuate in the hours and days after injury. There is evidence that some biomarkers correlate with—and can predict—outcome, though this may not be the case for all biomarkers, and specific roles remain to be clarified (Berger, 2006; Berger, Beers, Richichi, Wiesman, & Adelson, 2007; Chiaretti et al., 2008; Piazza, Storti, Cotena, Stoppa, et al., 2007). There is not yet consensus on which biomarker or combination thereof is the most useful. The brain biomarkers most thoroughly investigated to date include S100B, neuron-specific enolase (NSE), myelin basic protein (MBP), and glial fibrillary acid protein (GFAP; Sandler,

Child-SCAT3™ FIFA® ♀♀♀

Sport Concussion Assessment Tool for children ages 5 to 12 years
For use by medical professionals only

What is childSCAT3?[1]

The ChildSCAT3 is a standardized tool for evaluating injured children for concussion and can be used in children aged from 5 to 12 years. It supersedes the original SCAT and the SCAT2 published in 2005 and 2009, respectively[1]. For older persons, ages 13 years and over, please use the SCAT3. The ChildSCAT3 is designed for use by medical professionals. If you are not qualified, please use the Sport Concussion Recognition Tool[1]. Preseason baseline testing with the ChildSCAT3 can be helpful for interpreting post-injury test scores.

Specific instructions for use of the ChildSCAT3 are provided on page 3. If you are not familiar with the ChildSCAT3, please read through these instructions carefully. This tool may be freely copied in its current form for distribution to individuals, teams, groups and organizations. Any revision and any reproduction in a digital form require approval by the Concussion in Sport Group.
NOTE: The diagnosis of a concussion is a clinical judgment, ideally made by a medical professional. The ChildSCAT3 should not be used solely to make, or exclude, the diagnosis of concussion in the absence of clinical judgement. An athlete may have a concussion even if their ChildSCAT3 is "normal".

What is a concussion?

A concussion is a disturbance in brain function caused by a direct or indirect force to the head. It results in a variety of non-specific signs and/or symptoms (like those listed below) and most often does not involve loss of consciousness. Concussion should be suspected in the presence of any one or more of the following.

- Symptoms (e.g., headache), or
- Physical signs (e.g., unsteadiness), or
- Impaired brain function (e.g. confusion) or
- Abnormal behaviour (e.g., change in personality).

SIDELINE ASSESSMENT

Indications for Emergency Management

NOTE: A hit to the head can sometimes be associated with a more severe brain injury. If the concussed child displays any of the following, then do not proceed with the ChildSCAT3; instead activate emergency procedures and urgent transportation to the nearest hospital:

- Glasgow Coma score less than 15
- Deteriorating mental status
- Potential spinal injury
- Progressive, worsening symptoms or new neurologic signs
- Persistent vomiting
- Evidence of skull fracture
- Post traumatic seizures
- Coagulopathy
- History of Neurosurgery (eg Shunt)
- Multiple injuries

⒈ Glasgow coma scale (GCS)

Best eye response (E)

No eye opening	1
Eye opening in response to pain	2
Eye opening to speech	3
Eyes opening spontaneously	4

Best verbal response (V)

No verbal response	1
Incomprehensible sounds	2
Inappropriate words	3
Confused	4
Oriented	5

Best motor response (M)

No motor response	1
Extension to pain	2
Abnormal flexion to pain	3
Flexion/Withdrawal to pain	4
Localizes to pain	5
Obeys commands	6

Glasgow Coma score (E + V + M)	of 15

GCS should be recorded for all athletes in case of subsequent deterioration.

Potential signs of concussion?

If any of the following signs are observed after a direct or indirect blow to the head, the child should stop participation, be evaluated by a medical professional and **should not be permitted to return to sport the same day** if a concussion is suspected.

Any loss of consciousness?	Y	N
"If so, how long?"		
Balance or motor incoordination (stumbles, slow/laboured movements, etc.)?	Y	N
Disorientation or confusion (inability to respond appropriately to questions)?	Y	N
Loss of memory:	Y	N
"If so, how long?"		
"Before or after the injury?"		
Blank or vacant look:	Y	N
Visible facial injury in combination with any of the above:	Y	N

⒉ Sideline Assessment – child-Maddocks Score[3]

"I am going to ask you a few questions, please listen carefully and give your best effort."
Modified Maddocks questions (1 point for each correct answer)

Where are we at now?	0	1
Is it before or after lunch?	0	1
What did you have last lesson/class?	0	1
What is your teacher's name?	0	1
child-Maddocks score		of 4

Child-Maddocks score is for sideline diagnosis of concussion only and is not used for serial testing.

Any child with a suspected concussion should be REMOVED FROM PLAY, medically assessed and monitored for deterioration (i.e., should not be left alone). No child diagnosed with concussion should be returned to sports participation on the day of injury.

BACKGROUND

Name:	Date/Time of Injury:	
Examiner:	Date of Assessment:	
Sport/team/school:		
Age:	Gender:	M F
Current school year/grade:		
Dominant hand:	right	left neither
Mechanism of Injury ("tell me what happened"?):		

For Parent/carer to complete:

How many concussions has the child had in the past?		
When was the most recent concussion?		
How long was the recovery from the most recent concussion?		
Has the child ever been hospitalized or had medical imaging done (CT or MRI) for a head injury?	Y	N
Has the child ever been diagnosed with headaches or migraines?	Y	N
Does the child have a learning disability, dyslexia, ADD/ADHD, seizure disorder?	Y	N
Has the child ever been diagnosed with depression, anxiety or other psychiatric disorder?	Y	N
Has anyone in the family ever been diagnosed with any of these problems?	Y	N
Is the child on any medications? If yes, please list:	Y	N

FIGURE 4.1 Excerpt from the Child-SCAT3 Sport Concussion Assessment Tool.

Source: From Anon, (2015). Reprinted with permission of BMJ Publishing Group.

<table>
<tr><td>

SYMPTOM EVALUATION

3 Child report

Name:

	never	rarely	sometimes	often
I have trouble paying attention	0	1	2	3
I get distracted easily	0	1	2	3
I have a hard time concentrating	0	1	2	3
I have problems remembering what people tell me	0	1	2	3
I have problems following directions	0	1	2	3
I daydream too much	0	1	2	3
I get confused	0	1	2	3
I forget things	0	1	2	3
I have problems finishing things	0	1	2	3
I have trouble figuring things out	0	1	2	3
It's hard for me to learn new things	0	1	2	3
I have headaches	0	1	2	3
I feel dizzy	0	1	2	3
I feel like the room is spinning	0	1	2	3
I feel like I'm going to faint	0	1	2	3
Things are blurry when I look at them	0	1	2	3
I see double	0	1	2	3
I feel sick to my stomach	0	1	2	3
I get tired a lot	0	1	2	3
I get tired easily	0	1	2	3

Total number of symptoms (Maximum possible 20)
Symptom severity score (Maximum possible 20 x 3 = 60)

self rated   clinician interview   self rated and clinician monitored

4 Parent report

The child

	never	rarely	sometimes	often
has trouble sustaining attention	0	1	2	3
Is easily distracted	0	1	2	3
has difficulty concentrating	0	1	2	3
has problems remembering what he/she is told	0	1	2	3
has difficulty following directions	0	1	2	3
tends to daydream	0	1	2	3
gets confused	0	1	2	3
is forgetful	0	1	2	3
has difficulty completeing tasks	0	1	2	3
has poor problem solving skills	0	1	2	3
has problems learning	0	1	2	3
has headaches	0	1	2	3
feels dizzy	0	1	2	3
has a feeling that the room is spinning	0	1	2	3
feels faint	0	1	2	3
has blurred vision	0	1	2	3
has double vision	0	1	2	3
experiences nausea	0	1	2	3
gets tired a lot	0	1	2	3
gets tired easily	0	1	2	3

Total number of symptoms (Maximum possible 20)
Symptom severity score (Maximum possible 20 x 3 = 60)

Do the symptoms get worse with physical activity?   Y   N
Do the symptoms get worse with mental activity?   Y   N

parent self rated   clinician interview   parent self rated and clinician monitored

Overall rating for parent/teacher/coach/carer to answer.
How different is the child acting compared to his/her usual self?
Please circle one response:

no different   very different   unsure   N/A

Name of person completing Parent-report:
Relationship to child of person completing Parent-report:

Scoring on the ChildSCAT3 should not be used as a stand-alone method to diagnose concussion, measure recovery or make decisions about an athlete's readiness to return to competition after concussion.

</td><td>

COGNITIVE & PHYSICAL EVALUATION

5 Cognitive assessment
Standardized Assessment of Concussion – Child Version (SAC-C)[4]

Orientation (1 point for each correct answer)

What month is it?	0	1
What is the date today?	0	1
What is the day of the week?	0	1
What year is it?	0	1

Orientation score   of 4

Immediate memory

List	Trial 1	Trial 2	Trial 3	Alternative word list		
elbow	0 1	0 1	0 1	candle	baby	finger
apple	0 1	0 1	0 1	paper	monkey	penny
carpet	0 1	0 1	0 1	sugar	perfume	blanket
saddle	0 1	0 1	0 1	sandwich	sunset	lemon
bubble	0 1	0 1	0 1	wagon	iron	insect
Total						

Immediate memory score total   of 15

Concentration: Digits Backward

List	Trial 1	Alternative digit list		
6-2	0 1	5-2	4-1	4-9
4-9-3	0 1	6-2-9	5-2-6	4-1-5
3-8-1-4	0 1	3-2-7-9	1-7-9-5	4-9-6-8
6-2-9-7-1	0 1	1-5-2-8-6	3-8-5-2-7	6-1-8-4-3
7-1-8-4-6-2	0 1	5-3-9-1-4-8	8-3-1-9-6-4	7-2-4-8-5-6
Total of 5				

Concentration: Days in Reverse Order (1 pt. for entire sequence correct)

Sunday-Saturday-Friday-Thursday-Wednesday-Tuesday-Monday   0   1

Concentration score   of 6

6 Neck Examination:
Range of motion   Tenderness   Upper and lower limb sensation & strength
Findings:

7 Balance examination
Do one or both of the following tests.
Footwear (shoes, barefoot, braces, tape, etc.)

Modified Balance Error Scoring System (BESS) testing[5]
Which foot was tested (i.e. which is the **non-dominant** foot)   Left   Right
Testing surface (hard floor, field, etc.)
Condition
Double leg stance: Errors
Tandem stance (non-dominant foot at back):   Errors

Tandem gait[6,7]
Time to complete (best of 4 trials):   seconds
If child attempted, but unable to complete tandem gait, mark here

8 Coordination examination
Upper limb coordination
Which arm was tested: Left   Right
Coordination score   of 1

9 SAC Delayed Recall[4]
Delayed recall score   of 5

Since signs and symptoms may evolve over time, it is important to consider repeat evaluation in the acute assessment of concussion.

</td></tr>
</table>

FIGURE 4.1 (Continued)

Figaji, & Adelson, 2010). Children with mild TBI who typically have no radiological evidence of injury may especially benefit from biomarker assessment for prediction of brain injury severity and presence of secondary injury.

Caution is indicated in generalizing conclusions from adult TBI research on neurospecific biomarkers. There are known differences in pathophysiology between adults and children sustaining TBI, because of the unique biochemical, molecular, and cellular changes induced in young, fragile brains. Consequently, there are also differences in biomarker release during injury. In a similar vein, there is increasing support for differentiation of inflicted and accidental pediatric TBI on the basis of distinct biomarkers (Berger et al., 2006; Berger, Kochanek, & Pierce, 2004; Berger, Ta'asan, Rand, Lokshin, & Kochanek, 2009). Biomarker assessment may have particular benefits for inflicted TBI, where trauma history is often absent or inaccurate.

Conclusions

This chapter has provided some description of the standard tools used in clinical practice, as well as measures more commonly used or emerging in research settings. Tools are chosen to tap into areas that are vulnerable during the acute stage of recovery, assessing functions that have immediate and long-term impact on outcomes.

5

NEUROIMAGING IN CHILD TBI

Documentation of head and intracranial injury via neuroimaging is a core component of acute TBI assessment, as well as long-term follow-up. Although not specific to pediatric TBI, the National Institute of Neurological Disorders and Stroke (NINDS) makes neuroimaging recommendations as part of the TBI Common Data Elements, including proposed standardized imaging protocols, pathoanatomic terminology, and an overview of common imaging methods (Duhaime, Gean, Haacke, Hicks, et al., 2010, see also www.commondataelements.ninds.nih.gov/TBI.aspx; Haacke et al., 2010).

Though the physical and mathematical principles behind neuroimaging techniques are generally the same for adults and children, a number of modality-related strengths and weaknesses need to be considered when imaging the child TBI population. Among these are considerations for 1) imaging protocol length, as children may find it difficult to remain still for the required amount of time, and motion artifact may significantly reduce the quality and resolution of the images; 2) sedation and anesthesia-related medical risks and complications for those too young or too agitated to undergo scanning procedures awake; 3) minimizing ionizing radiation, which can increase the risk of cancer, especially in very young children; 4) sensitivity of particular techniques to non-accidental trauma; and 5) usefulness of particular techniques in preverbal children, in whom injury assessment is more difficult.

In addition, general neuroimaging guidelines for pediatric populations should be considered. Clinical scanning for TBI is usually conducted in urgent situations, precluding the possibility of familiarization; however, the use of a mock scanner is recommended prior to research scanning, or in other diagnostic situations, because it can improve the quality of both structural and functional scans, eliminate the need for sedation, increase compliance, and reduce anxiety (de Amorim e Silva, Mackenzie, Hallowell, Stewart, & Ditchfield, 2006; de Bie, Boersma, Wat-tjes, Adriaanse, et al., 2010; Epstein, Casey, Tonev, Davidson, et al., 2007; Raschle, Lee, Buechler, Christodoulou, et al., 2009; Tyc, Fairclough, Fletcher, Leigh, & Mulhern, 1995). Other preparative approaches and guidelines, such as play ther-apy (Pressdee, May, Eastman, & Grier, 1997), feeding and behavioral training (Raschle et al., 2012; Raschle et al., 2009; Slifer, Bucholtz, & Cataldo, 1994; Slifer, Koontz, & Cataldo, 2002), video training (Slifer, 1996), and simulation (Rosen-berg, Sweeney, Gillen, Kim, et al., 1997) may also be helpful in reducing motion artifacts and for the child's well-being. Specific recommendations and guidelines have been developed for functional magnetic resonance imaging (fMRI) scan-ning, which tends to be lengthy and more often used for research (Byars, Holland, Strawsburg, Bommer, et al., 2002; Kotsoni, Byrd, & Casey, 2006; Wilke, Holland, Myseros, Schmithorst, & Ball, 2003).

Neuroimaging techniques have advanced rapidly in the last two decades, and there are ever-increasing choices to consider for determining both the structural and functional consequences of TBI on the developing brain. An understanding of the pathophysiology and types of damage likely to occur after child TBI can be useful in determining type and timing of various neuroimaging modalities. TBI lesions can occur anywhere in the brain and can affect the skull itself through fractures; thus, divergent imaging techniques may be more suitable to particular lesions (e.g., subdural, cortical, subcortical), mechanisms (e.g., accidental vs. non-accidental TBI), and also to particular age ranges (children under the age of 2, school-age children, adolescents).

Conventional Neuroimaging Techniques

Plain Film Radiography

Radiography, which uses a beam of X-rays, is one of the oldest imaging techniques. In radiography of the head, a portion of these rays are absorbed, depending on the composition and density of brain structures and regions; the remaining portion of the X-ray is then captured by a detector once it has passed through the head, yielding a two-dimensional representation of the scanned structures. Compared to computed tomography (CT), cranial radiography uses much less radiation, making it a viable alternative in that regard. However, despite its good sensitivity for detection of skull fractures, it is not sensitive enough for the detection of intracranial lesions and is therefore not widely used, as a negative X-ray does not exclude the possibility of intracranial pathology in at-risk patients. There are, however, some exceptions to this, particularly in young children, in whom it may be beneficial to optimize radiography use to balance the increased radiation dangers associated with CT (see below). Radiography can also play a role in preventing rare complications associated with skull fractures, such as leptomeningeal cysts. A number of protocols and preliminary attempts at developing clinical decision rules for the use of radiography have been proposed based on expert opinion groups; however, these have not been validated, remain imprecise, or are not clinically useful, although work is currently underway to refine such rules (Beaudin, Saint-Vil, Ouimet, Mercier, & Crevier, 2007; Bin, Schutzman, & Greenes, 2010; Browning, Reed, Wilkinson, & Beattie, 2005).

Computed Tomography (CT)

CT is the most widely used technique for acute assessment of head trauma and associated brain injuries. The principle behind the technique is similar to that of radiography, utilizing ionizing radiation with detectors to produce images of the skull and brain, based on tissue attenuation of X-rays. In many ways, it is ideal for acute imaging in children because it is readily accessible in the emergency department, relatively inexpensive, and easy to use. It also has a short acquisition time compared to other structural imaging modalities, which is a significant advantage in young children, who may not tolerate lengthy protocols during which they are required to be immobile and confined to a small space. CT is especially useful in providing information for acute clinical decision making because it can rapidly detect lesions that may require immediate medical intervention, such as depressed skull fractures or large hematomas that can displace brain structures or raise intracranial pressure, necessitating neurosurgical intervention. CT scanning is also sensitive to skull fractures, which may overlie intraparenchymal injuries. Serial CT is often used to track lesion progression in the initial hours or days following the injury and is especially useful for severe TBI, in which rapid deterioration in mental state can indicate developing intracranial pathology not initially seen on acute CT.

On one hand, CT can be useful in evaluating the consequence of head injury in preverbal children, because they are difficult to assess using standardized tools and significant brain injury can consequently go undetected (Schutzman, Barnes, Duhaime, Greenes, et al., 2001). On the other hand, the technique has come under intense scrutiny, especially for young children with mild forms of head injury, due to increasing concerns related to the amount of radiation absorbed by children during the scan and the risks and morbidity associated with radiation (Brenner, Elliston, Hall, & Berdon, 2001) and sedation (Conners, Sacks, & Leahey, 1999; Vade, Sukhani, Dolenga, & Habisohn-Schuck, 1995). Though the rate varies according to age, dose and body location, it is clear that the lifetime risk of developing cancer after a single CT is much greater for young children compared to older children and adults (D. J. Brenner, 2010; Hall, 2002). This has led to a number of multicenter efforts to define clinical decision-making algorithms guiding CT use and determining when it can be deferred (Dunning, Daly, Lomas, Lecky, et al., 2006; Kuppermann, Holmes,

Dayan, Hoyle, et al., 2009; Osmond, Klassen, Wells, Correll, et al., 2010). Among its other downsides compared to alternative techniques, such as magnetic resonance imaging (MRI), are its relatively poorer spatial resolution and more limited ability to detect diffuse axonal injury (DAI).

Magnetic Resonance Imaging (MRI)

MRI uses a magnetic field strength to align atoms in the body. Radio-frequency pulses are emitted to alter this alignment, causing nuclei to produce a rotating magnetic field detected by the scanner and then reconstructed into images. MRI is considered to be superior to CT in detecting more subtle lesions, and this sensitivity improves with increasing magnetic field strength (e.g., 1.5 vs. 3 tesla). Its capacity to detect some lesions that are not seen on CT suggests it can increase diagnostic accuracy, while reducing radiation risk in pediatric TBI (e.g., Lee, Wintermark, Gean, Ghajar, et al., 2008; see also Suskauer & Huisman, 2009).

A number of standard sequences are typically used in evaluating the neuroanatomical consequences of TBI, with each capitalizing on the properties of different tissue types. T1-weighted images provide good contrast between gray and white matter because they differentiate fat (bright signal) from water (dark signal). T2-weighted images are also included in standard protocols and are also sensitive to fat/water differentiation, though the contrast in the case of T2 is inverse (water is brighter). T2 images are based on spin echo sequences. Fluid-attenuated inversion recovery (FLAIR) images are based on T2-weighted imaging, in which fluid (e.g., cerebrospinal fluid) is suppressed (or "nulled") to bring out the effects of lesions in periventricular regions. FLAIR is therefore useful for detecting nonhemorrhagic cortical contusions, subdural hemorrhages, and diffuse axonal injury (DAI). Gradient-recalled echo (GRE, T2* or fast field echo), like T1 and T2, is a pulse sequence. Unlike T1 and T2, which are useful for the detection of subacute and chronic bleeds, it is more sensitive to hyperacute parenchymal blood because of its sensitivity to static magnetic inhomogeneity.

Despite MRI's superior spatial resolution and ability to offer a variety of lesion detection sequences leading to greater sensitivity, CT is more frequently used in clinical neuroimaging because of its accessibility and speed. CT is also more readily accessible to patients who may have contraindications to MRI scanning because of the presence of a high magnetic field (e.g., metallic implants, dental braces). Nonetheless, MRI is a frequent tool of clinical practice, especially when clinical symptomatology is not explained by CT findings, suggesting undetected lesions (e.g., DAI). Its utility in settings where the timing of scanning is not constrained by clinical management requirements, such as in TBI follow-up (subacute or chronic stages) or research settings, is greatly increased. See figures 5.1 and 5.2 for representative examples of CT and MRI scanning results after pediatric TBI.

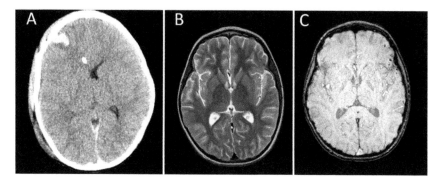

FIGURE 5.1 Results of (A) CT, (B) T2-weighted MRI, and (C) SWI images for a male patient (8.5 years) with TBI at equivalent anatomical levels. His GCS on presentation to the ED was 8. The CT demonstrates right intraparenchymal contusions and small amounts of extra axial haemorrhage. The T2-weighted MRI shows right frontal and temporal gray matter and white matter haemorrhage and gliosis. The SWI scan shows additional multifocal regions of haemorrhage in the frontal lobes and right multifocal parietal gray matter signal loss.

Source: From Beauchamp et al. (2011). Reprinted with permission of Mary Ann.

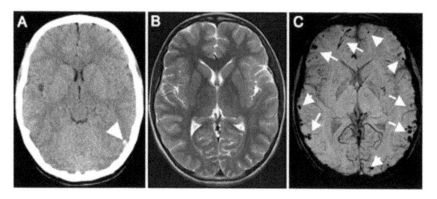

FIGURE 5.2 Results of (A) CT, (B) T2-weighted MRI, and (C) SWI images for a male patient (10.9 years) with TBI at equivalent anatomical levels. His GCS on presentation to the ED was 13. The CT demonstrates a focus of hemorrhage in the left occipital lobe (arrowhead). The same lesion is poorly seen on the T2-weighted MRI; however, SWI demonstrates multiple foci of hemorhage (arrows) not identified on the other scans.

Source: Liebert Publishing.

Electroencephalography (EEG)

Electroencephalography records the electrical activity of neurons in the brain using multiple electrodes placed at predetermined locations on the scalp. Electrical brain activity fluctuates as a function of time, and, when stimuli are introduced, their cerebral processing is reflected in changes in electric field potentials, which provide clinicians with information on normal and abnormal brain activity (Wallace, Wagner, Wagner, & McDeavitt, 2001).

In child TBI, EEG and amplitude EEG are useful mainly in two clinical contexts. First, EEG can be used continuously to detect or monitor brain activity in the case of post-injury coma or vegetative state. In cases in which children experience a prolonged period of unconsciousness following TBI, it may be necessary for medical decision making and for evaluation of prognosis to distinguish between coma (in which patients are in a state of deep unconsciousness, lack wakefulness, and are completely unaware of themselves or their environment), vegetative state (in which patients are unaware of themselves or their environment, but alternate between periods of intermittent wakefulness and unconsciousness as manifested by sleep-wake cycles), and brain death (in which patients lack wakefulness and awareness and have deficient brain-stem function, preventing them from independent respiratory regulation). The most common EEG finding in vegetative state is that of diffuse generalized polymorphic delta or theta wave activity; alpha rhythms, on the other hand, may appear and increase as level of consciousness improves (e.g., minimally conscious state) (Ashwal, 2004).

Second, EEG can be used acutely or long-term for detecting post-traumatic epilepsy, a seizure disorder caused by traumatic injury to the brain. In general terms, acute post-TBI epilepsy is fairly frequent and occurs in approximately 15% of patients with severe injuries, whereas those with mild injuries have a risk level comparable to that of the general population. It is slightly less common in children with severe TBI (about 10%) (Herman, 2002). Risk factors for post-traumatic seizures include young age (0–3 years), length of loss of consciousness and PTA, penetrating injury, non-accidental injury, parenchymal injury, depressed skull fractures, and, especially, diffuse cerebral contusions and subdural hematomas (Agrawal, Timothy, Pandit, & Manju, 2006; Arango, Deibert, Brown, Bell, et al., 2012). Late seizures are less frequent, as is the development of full-blown epilepsy, though a proportion of children will go on to develop chronic post-TBI epilepsy (recurrent unprovoked seizures), and those with early seizures are more likely to experience late seizures (Emanuelson & Uvebrant, 2009).

Advanced and Experimental Neuroimaging Techniques

Neuroimaging is a rapidly evolving field, and new techniques or specialized analysis methodologies are constantly changing the face of clinical practice and research in children with TBI. The controversy surrounding radiation risk associated with CT scanning in children, as well as the observation in a number of studies that injury characteristics detected on CT and MRI do not necessarily correlate with neuropsychological outcomes, have also contributed to the emergence of alternative imaging options. At the mild end of the TBI spectrum, documentation of inconsistencies between pathology detection (or lack thereof) and clinical or neuropsychological outcome has been spurred by the capabilities of more sensitive structural and functional imaging techniques. Mild TBI was previously thought to have innocuous neurological consequences; however, there is now evidence that it can be associated with both structural lesions often invisible on conventional CT and functional disturbances (e.g., microhemorrhages, abnormal metabolism, reduced blood flow, impaired neural transmission) detectable only using cutting-edge functional techniques (Beauchamp, Ditchfield, Babl, Kean, et al., 2011; Ewing-Cobbs, Prasad, Kramer, Louis, et al., 2000; MacKenzie, Siddiqi, Babb, Bagley, et al., 2002; Povlishock, 1993; Umile, Sandel, Alavi, Terry, & Plotkin, 2002; Wozniak, Krach, Ward, Mueller, et al., 2007). Some emerging techniques may require access to new and complex infrastructure or to advanced, time-consuming analysis capabilities; others take advantage of the properties of readily available technology (e.g., MRI). As a result, not all techniques presented here are suitable or feasible for the clinical assessment of TBI, but many are already frequently used in the context of TBI research and can inform clinical practice. Published reviews of many of these techniques are available (Belanger, Vanderploeg, Curtiss, & Warden, 2007; Coles, 2007; Gallagher, Hutchinson, & Pickard, 2007; Hillary, Steffener, Biswal, Lange, et al., 2002; Hunter, Wilde, Tong, & Holshouser, 2012; Kou, Wu, Tong, Holshouser, et al., 2010; Tshibanda, Vanhaudenhuyse, Boly, Soddu, et al., 2009; Van Boven, Harrington, Hackney, Ebel, et al., 2009), with some specific to child TBI (Ashwal, Holshouser, & Tong, 2006; Suskauer & Huisman, 2009.

MRI-Based Techniques

Diffusion weighted/tensor imaging (DWI/DTI) + apparent diffusion coefficient mapping. DWI is a MRI-based technique that takes advantage of the characteristics of water diffusion within brain tissue to produce in vivo structural images. DWI assesses the manner in which water diffuses through the brain and is therefore sensitive to edema. Through this property it can also detect ischemia and DAI. Similarly, DTI allows the reproduction of neural tracts in the brain by measuring the restriction of water diffusion in tissue. Water molecules in the brain are known to move quickly when parallel to nerve fibers rather than perpendicular to them (anisotropic diffusion). This characteristic is determined by the thickness of the myelin surrounding the axons, yielding a variable called fractional anisotropy. DWI and DTI are unique in their capability to quantify, detect, and visualize white-matter changes. In TBI, changes in diffusivity or anisotropy are used as indicators of structural alterations that may result from damage or degeneration of white-matter fibers through breakdown of myelin and nerve terminals, or neuronal swelling or shrinkage (see figures 5.3 and 5.4) (Ducreux, Huynh, Fillard, Renoux, et al., 2005). This makes the technique particularly useful in the detection of axonal injury in white matter (Wozniak et al., 2007). Initially used in case studies of pediatric TBI, its unique capabilities for detection of white-matter injury have since made DTI especially useful in child TBI for assessing the integrity of the corpus callosum (Babikian, Marion, Copeland, Alger, et al., 2010; Ewing-Cobbs, Prasad, Swank, Kramer, et al., 2008; Wilde, McCauley, Hunter, Bigler,

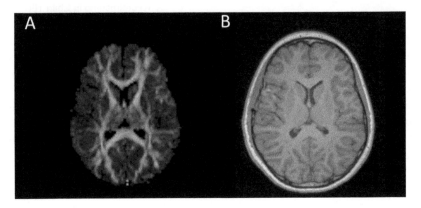

FIGURE 5.3 Functional anisotropy map (A) for a 12.5 year old boy who sustained a moderate TBI (GCS 10) in a motor vehicle accident. Structural T-1 weighted MRI (B) showed severe right posterior frontal and temporal hemorrhage and associated enchephalomacia.

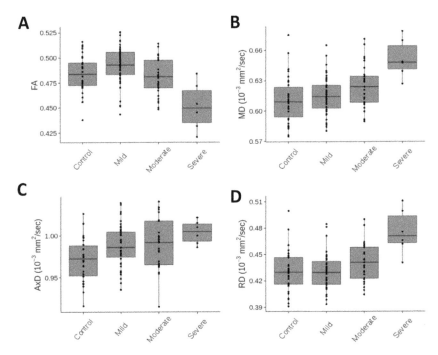

FIGURE 5.4 Illustration of DTI metrics across TBI severity levels. Imaging was performed on average 30 days post-injury in 78 children with TBI and 30 healthy controls (age range 6–16 years).

In these groups, all four diffusion metrics were significantly altered in the severe TBI group compared with controls.

(A) Fractional anisotropy (FA) is a marker of white matter microstructure. Decreases in functional anisotropy may indicate white matter damage or loss; (B) An increase in mean diffusivity (MD) may indicate white matter loss; (C) An increase in axial diffusivity (AxD) combined with axonal injury and an increase in (D) radial diffusivity (RD) may indicate loss of myelination.

et al., 2008; Wu, Wilde, Bigler, Merkley, et al., 2010). The technique also shows good correlation with injury severity (Benson, Meda, Vasudevan, Kou, et al., 2007; Wilde, Newsome, Bigler, Pertab, et al., 2011; Yuan, Holland, Schmithorst, Walz, et al., 2007) and neuropsychological, social, and functional outcomes (e.g., Ewing-Cobbs et al., 2008; Hanten, Wilde, Menefee, Li, et al., 2008; Levin, Wilde, Chu, Yallampalli, et al., 2008; McCauley, Wilde, Bigler, Chu, et al., 2011; Wozniak et al., 2007). A disadvantage of DTI, particularly in pediatric populations, is that the sequence produces a loud noise that can be disturbing to children. In addition, though the acquisition of more diffusion directions increases the quality of DTI data, it can also considerably lengthen scanning times and therefore be more susceptible to motion artifacts in children.

Susceptibility weighted imaging (SWI). SWI is a specific MRI sequence that exploits the magnetic susceptibility differences between tissues and is therefore useful for identifying extravascular blood products (Haacke, Xu, Cheng, & Reichenbach, 2004). In the context of brain trauma, SWI has been reported to significantly increase lesion detection, depicting up to six times as many lesions and double the apparent volume of hemorrhagic lesions (Tong, Ashwal, Holshouser, Shutter, et al., 2003). SWI is therefore one of the most promising sequences for use in the field of TBI. SWI's increased sensitivity to blood products makes it particularly useful for the detection of microhemorrhages, the presence of which has been shown to be related to poor outcome in children with non-accidental brain trauma (Colbert, Holshouser, Aaen, Sheridan, et al., 2010). Studies evaluating the effectiveness of the technique in children have reported its value in detecting small, diffuse lesions, such as those typical of traumatic (or diffuse) axonal injury (Sigmund, Tong, Nickerson, Wall, et al., 2007; Tong, Ashwal, Holshouser, Nickerson, et al., 2004; Tong et al., 2003). In a prospective study of all child TBI severity types, Beauchamp and colleagues (Beauchamp, Ditchfield, Babl, Kean, et al., 2011) found that SWI detected lesions more frequently than CT or conventional MRI sequences and was also useful in identifying additional or multifocal lesions not otherwise seen on CT or conventional MRI (see figures 5.1 and 5.2). Its superiority in lesion detection is well supported, and evidence of a relationship between the presence of SWI lesions and clinical and neuropsychological outcomes is emerging. Initial studies indicate correlations between SWI lesion number/volume and clinical (e.g., GCS) and cognitive (e.g., IQ) outcomes (Babikian, Freier, Tong, Nickerson, et al., 2005; Beauchamp, Beare, Ditchfield, Coleman, et al., 2013; Colbert et al., 2010; Tong et al., 2004). Like other MRI techniques, SWI is susceptible to artifacts at air-tissue interfaces (e.g., sinuses), often compromising visualization of the orbitofrontal areas of the brain.

Magnetic resonance spectroscopy (MRS). Proton MRS (1H-MRS) measures the relative concentration of metabolites (e.g., NAA, creatine, cystolic choline compounds) in a given volume of brain tissue using spectroscopic analysis (Rigotti, Inglese, & Gonen, 2007) and thus may provide additional neuropathological information that may be useful in determining prognosis after child TBI. For example, N-acetylaspartate (NAA), an amino acid that acts as a neuronal marker, is reduced when neurons are damaged or lose function after TBI. Correlations between specific metabolite reductions and neuropsychological and behavioral function are reported after child TBI (Ashwal, Babikian, Gardner-Nichols, Freier, et al., 2006; Ashwal, Holshouser, Tong, Serna, et al., 2004; Babikian et al., 2005; Brenner, Freier, Holshouser, Burley, & Ashwal, 2003; Hunter, Thornton, Wang, Levin, et al., 2005; Yeo, Phillips, Jung, Brown, et al., 2006). MRS is promising in child TBI, because it may be useful in differentiating between non-accidental and accidental brain injury (Aaen, Holshouser, Sheridan, Colbert, et al., 2010; Holshouser, Ashwal, Luh, Shu, et al., 1997). In addition, because of its sensitivity to neurochemical alterations, it may provide information on significant brain changes that correlate with functional outcomes in otherwise normal-appearing brains (Garnett, Blamire, Corkill, Cadoux-Hudson, et al., 2000; Holshouser, Tong, & Ashwal, 2005). As with DTI, interpretation of MRS data requires expertise in post-processing and analysis of the images, and it may therefore not be accessible in clinical contexts.

Functional MRI (fMRI) and functional connectivity. Functional MRI uses the blood-oxygen-level dependent (BOLD) technique to measure cerebral activity, often in response to stimulation, and is based on the principle that deoxyhemoglobin has greater magnetic susceptibility than oxyhemoglobin. Changes in oxy- and deoxy-hemoglobin and their corresponding paramagnetic/diamagnetic properties are recorded as a proxy for brain blood flow (T2* acquisition sequences are used). To date, fMRI has not been incorporated into clinical practice, though results from a number of studies suggest it can be useful for diagnostic purposes as well as for evaluation of outcome (see Munson, Schroth, & Ernst, 2006). The technique is mainly used experimentally to answer specific task-related questions using paradigms to evoke brain activity responses to cognitive, sensory, or motor stimuli. It has the same advantages as structural MRI in terms of its superior spatial resolution and absence of radiation. In children with TBI, fMRI has been used to document alterations in brain activity, including compensatory motor functioning (Caeyenberghs, Wenderoth, Smits-Engelsman, Sunaert, & Swinnen, 2009), as well as neural processing of attention, working memory (Kramer, Chiu, Walz, Holland, et al., 2008; Newsome, Scheibel, Hunter, Wang, et al., 2007), and language networks (Karunanayaka, Holland, Yuan, Altaye, et al., 2007). The clinical use of fMRI is currently limited by the considerable expertise and time required for data analysis, making it less suitable for clinical practice. Restrictions exist for its use in very young children because of the necessity to lie still in the scanner during activation paradigms.

An additional feature of fMRI is the possibility of conducting studies of the brain "at rest," which can provide information on functional organization and connectivity between brain regions via resting-state-networks (see Freilich & Gaillard, 2010; Rosazza & Minati, 2011; van den Heuvel & Hulshoff Pol, 2010; Vogel, Power, Petersen, & Schlaggar, 2010). The technique has been applied to adults with TBI (e.g., Hillary, Slocomb, Hills, Fitzpatrick, et al., 2011; Kasahara, Menon,

Salmond, Outtrim, et al., 2010; Marquez de la Plata, Garces, Shokri Kojori, Grinnan, et al., 2011; Mayer, Mannell, Ling, Gasparovic, & Yeo, 2011), and it is thought that the technique holds promise for understanding recovery and the impact of therapeutic interventions on default functioning of the brain after injury (Hunter et al., 2012). Studies are likely to emerge in pediatric TBI populations over the coming years, because the technique is relatively easy to implement in participants undergoing fMRI activation studies.

Quantitative methods for structural MRI. There are a number of post-processing analytic methods that can provide quantitative information on brain structure based on data acquired using structural MRI. Widespread techniques, including volumetrics or voxel-based morphometry (VBM), are based on voxel-by-voxel comparisons (either manual or automated) of gray matter, white matter, and cerebrospinal fluid, providing information on the structural integrity of regions of interest in the brain. Certain software for post-processing analysis also permits calculations of cortical thickness in the brain. These techniques have been used extensively in children with TBI, revealing both diffuse volumetric changes in the brain (e.g., Bigler, Abildskov, Wilde, McCauley, et al., 2010; Tasker, Salmond, Westland, Pena, et al., 2005; Wilde et al., 2005) and atrophy in specific regions of vulnerability, such as the corpus callosum, hippocampus, amygdala, and cerebellum (e.g., Beauchamp, Anderson, Catroppa, Maller, et al., 2009; Beauchamp, Anderson, et al., 2011; Spanos, Wilde, Bigler, Cleavinger, et al., 2007; Wilde, Bigler, Hunter, Fearing, et al., 2007), as well as reduced cortical thickness (see Figure 5.5) (e.g., Merkley et al., 2008).

Near-Infrared Spectroscopy (NIRS)

NIRS is a functional, spectroscopic method that measures the wavelength and intensity of the absorption of near-infrared light by tissue and is based on overtone and combination vibrations. The technique is relatively noninvasive and can be used to assess brain function by detecting changes in hemoglobin levels associated with neural activity by shining an infrared light through the skull. NIRS has the advantage of being much more portable than other functional neuroimaging techniques and less sensitive to motion artifacts. This is a significant advantage in infants and young children, who are difficult to assess using CT or MRI without sedation. In the context of TBI, NIRS may be used for a variety of functions, including monitoring of cerebral oxygenation (Haitsma & Maas, 2007; Tachtsidis, Tisdall, Pritchard, Leung, et al., 2011) and hemodynamic changes that may be related to diffuse swelling or other pathology (Adelson, Nemoto, Colak, & Painter, 1998). Handheld devices are beginning to be developed and show some promise for use in the initial examination and screening of patients for brain hematomas that may require urgent surgical treatment (Leon-Carrion, Dominguez-Roldan, Leon-Dominguez, & Murillo-Cabezas, 2010). The technique can also be used in a functional mode whereby stimuli (e.g., cognitive, language, visual, motor) are presented to subjects and brain activity

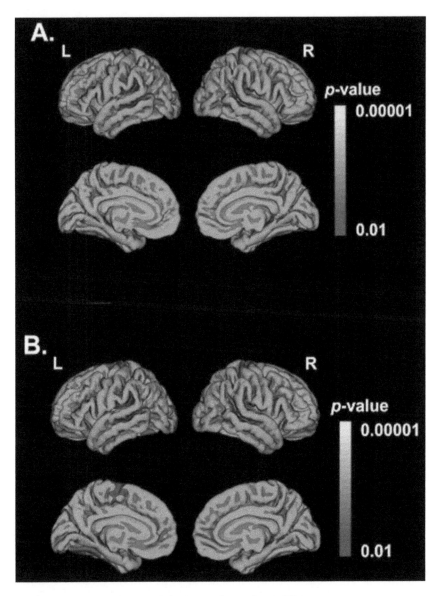

FIGURE 5.5 Changes in cortical thickness after pediatric TBI.

A–B: Between-group cortical thickness differences at 3-months (1A) and 18-months (1B) post-injury in 20 children with moderate-severe TBI. Blue regions indicate significantly thinner cerebral cortex in the trauamtic brain injury (TBI) group.

Source: From Wilde et al. (2012). Reprinted with permission of Elsevier.

in response to stimulation is recorded, though research in TBI populations is still in its infancy (Bhambhani, Maikala, Farag, & Rowland, 2006). The main disadvantage of the technique is that, to date, it can be used only to scan cortical tissue, because near-infrared light does not penetrate deep enough to reach subcortical structures.

Single Photon Emission Computed Tomography (SPECT) and Positron Emission Tomography (PET)

SPECT and PET scanning techniques are both based on the injection of radioactive tracer materials, which are taken up by brain tissue proportionally to cerebral blood flow and are therefore a direct measure of brain activity. As the tracer decays, it emits a photon (SPECT) or positron (PET), which is detected and localized. These nuclear medicine techniques have very little current application to the assessment and follow-up of child TBI, because the use of radiation significantly limits their appropriateness. The relatively high cost, long scanning times (dependent on the tracer used), and inaccessibility of the infrastructure further constrain their clinical application. Earlier studies in children aimed to monitor brain activity after rehabilitation, identifying functional lesions, as well as measuring cerebral activation, plasticity, and metabolites (e.g., Emanuelson, von Wendt, Bjure, Wiklund, & Uvebrant, 1997; Goshen, Zwas, Shahar, & Tadmor, 1996; Muller, Behen, Rothermel, Muzik, et al., 1999; Worley, Hoffman, Paine, Kalman, et al., 1995). In adults, they are considered useful for the study of neurometabolism and have been used to investigate post-traumatic neurotransmitters and metabolites that can be targeted by selection of the tracer used (e.g., Folkersma, Boellaard, Yaqub, Kloet, et al., 2011; Ostberg, Virta, Rinne, Oikonen, et al., 2011).

Magnetoencephalography (MEG)/Magnetic Source Imaging (MSI)

MEG records the magnetic fields emitted by electrical currents between synapses or in neurons. With this technique, real-time brain activity can be monitored. The data generated can be combined with data from MRI to localize the source of the brain activity and construct images of this activity (Magnetic Source Imaging, MSI). This provides an advantage of MEG over EEG, because precise temporal and spatial patterns can be observed. MEG may be useful in detecting subtle changes not seen with conventional imaging techniques (Bigler, 1999). Its clinical utility remains limited because of (a) restricted access to the technology in clinical centers, (b) the need for extensive training, and (c) time for the complex data analysis required. To date, it has been used in research settings to detect mild TBI in adults (Huang, Theilmann, Robb, Angeles, et al., 2009; Lewine, Davis, Sloan, Kodituwakku, & Orrison, 1999).

Typical Neuroanatomical Changes Following Pediatric TBI and Functional Implications

Using the varied techniques described earlier in this chapter, neuroimaging studies have extensively documented the types of primary and secondary neuropathology typical of childhood brain injuries (for example, see Pinto, Meoded, Poretti, Tekes, & Huisman, 2012, 2013). Besides providing critical diagnostic and descriptive information on the severity, type, location, and distribution of lesions in the brain, the identification of neuropathology using structural imaging techniques can inform the functional consequences of brain injury. The heterogeneity of lesions and distribution in the brain, as well as the diffuse nature of most injuries, often precludes exact localizationist correlations with function; however, MRI and SWI studies link structural and microstructural findings with cognitive and sociocognitive outcomes (e.g., Babikian et al., 2005; Beauchamp, Beare, et al., 2013; Ryan, Catroppa, Cooper, Beare, et al., 2015; Schmidt, Hanten, Li, Wilde, et al., 2013; Verger, Junque, Levin, Jurado, et al., 2001; Wilde, Hunter, & Bigler, 2012).

Neuroanatomical findings are diverse and are a function of injury severity, though a frontotemporal distribution is common (Beauchamp, Ditchfield, et al., 2011; Bigler, Abildskov, Petrie, Farrer, et al., 2013; Keightley, Sinopoli, Davis, Mikulis, et al., 2014; Wilde et al., 2005). The global consequences of these injuries can translate to overall brain atrophy, with reductions in brain volume observed in gray and white matter and reflected by enlarged ventricular volumes (Bigler, 1999; see Ross, 2011, for a review; Verger et al., 2001).

The use of diffusion tensor imaging (DTI) has enabled precise study of white-matter change (see Roberts, Mathias, & Rose, 2014, for a meta-analysis), with studies showing that white-matter integrity remains abnormal in children with TBI more than 12 months following the injury (Wilde et al., 2006; Wozniak et al., 2007; Yuan et al., 2007). White-matter changes are further reflected by changes in the integrity and appearance of the corpus callosum (Babikian et al., 2010; Beauchamp, Ditchfield, Catroppa, et al., 2011; Tasker, 2006; Wu et al., 2010) and functional associations with cognition, working memory, social cognition and skills, and motor function (Adamson, Yuan, Babcock, Leach, et al., 2013; Beauchamp et al., 2009; Caeyenberghs, Leemans, Geurts, Taymans, et al., 2010; Ewing-Cobbs et al., 2008; Kurowski, Wade, Cecil, Walz, et al., 2009; Levin, Wilde, et al., 2008; Wilde et al., 2011).

Studies focusing on particular regions of interest have shown marked reductions of hippocampal and cerebellar volumes (Spanos et al., 2007; Tasker et al., 2005; Wilde et al., 2007), suggesting these areas are particularly vulnerable to injury in children. Less attention has focused on limbic and deep nuclei structures, but evidence exists of amygdala and basal ganglia alterations in the long term after severe child TBI (Beauchamp, Ditchfield, Maller, et al., 2011; Wilde et al., 2007). Regional structural and functional changes have also been associated with poorer outcome in related cognitive domains, such as memory (Newsome, Scheibel, Steinberg, Troyanskaya, et al., 2007; Serra-Grabulosa, Junque, Verger, Salgado-Pineda, et al., 2005).

Conclusions

The field of neuroimaging provides a number of interesting structural and functional options for the detection and depiction of skull and brain changes related to pediatric TBI. To comprehensively assess the integrity of the developing brain, many of these are often used in combination, as each offers a variety of advantages for particular cerebral components. Though a number of advanced techniques can provide increased sensitivity and more detailed description of post-injury function and structure, the implementation of some of these techniques is somewhat limited by financial, time, and infrastructure considerations in clinical settings. However, rapid advancements in neuroimaging modalities, and improvements in the accessibility and ease of analysis for these techniques, continue to increase the possibilities for acute and long-term diagnosis and management of cranial and intracranial injuries related to pediatric TBI.

6

MULTIDISCIPLINARY ASSESSMENT FOLLOWING CHILD TBI

The evaluation of brain-behavior relationships is at the heart of post-TBI assessment practices and is useful regardless of the presence or extent of structural and functional lesions. The rapid progression of neuroimaging technology has made it increasingly possible to determine the location and severity of injury, to some extent facilitating predictions as to what type and range of neuropsychological deficits may be expected. In spite of these advances, outcome after child TBI remains difficult to predict because of large individual variations in performance, as well as the presence of numerous confounding factors (e.g., pre-morbid functioning, family environment, access to rehabilitation resources). In addition, outcome after TBI does not always follow predictable patterns in children, because injury occurs during a dynamic developmental period. As a result, inconsistencies in severity-outcome relationships are common (Fay, Yeates, Wade, Drotar, et al., 2009; Yeates, 2010). Such discrepancies may also be the result of neuroimaging limitations in detecting subtle structural and functional brain changes (e.g., small lesions not seen on conventional MRI, metabolic disturbances, functional changes in brain activity in the absence of structural damage, global brain atrophy measurable through quantitative methods, but not apparent on standard clinical imaging) (e.g., Beauchamp, Ditchfield, et al., 2011; Ewing-Cobbs et al., 2000; MacKenzie et al., 2002; Povlishock, 1993; Umile, Sandel, Alavi, Terry, & Plotkin, 2002; Wozniak et al., 2007). In addition, correlations between test performance and central nervous system damage may not be as clear in children, because their injuries tend to be diffuse and their cognitive functions are less localized than those of adults (e.g., Bigler et al., 2010; Ciesielski, Lesnik, Savoy, Grant, & Ahlfors, 2006). In a context of uncertain outcomes, the position of the neuropsychologist is central within the medical and allied health team and in relation to families, teachers, and other professionals. Neuropsychologists play a pivotal role in using mixed assessment methods (standardized testing, parent report, observation, projective testing) to provide information on a range of functions (e.g., cognitive, perceptual, motor, social, academic, adaptive, behavioral, psychological) that may be affected following the injury.

Principles of Neuropsychological Assessment After Child TBI

Many principles of adult neuropsychological assessment have driven the evolution of child neuropsychological assessment. However, there are just as many special considerations that must be taken into account to reflect the particularities of child assessment. These have been described in full in previous reference texts of developmental neuropsychology and are summarized here (Anderson, Northam, Hendy, & Wrennall, 2001; Baron, 2004; Yeates, Ris, Taylor, & Pennington, 2010). Neuropsychological evaluation of child TBI outcomes is anchored in these fundamental principles. However, further considerations need to be taken into account in tailoring neuropsychological testing to children with brain injury, as will be outlined in the following sections.

Dominating the list of assessment principles is the notion that child neuropsychological evaluation occurs in a dynamic maturational period and can therefore provide only a "snapshot" of a child's abilities at the time of testing. This is particularly true in the context of acquired brain injury, which perturbs the normal trajectory of rapid brain development. This has implications for determining a child's performance during the post-injury recovery period. The performance of children with TBI is usually compared to that of non-injured peers; however, the latter are themselves in a dynamic, nonlinear, and sometimes exponential period of cerebral and cognitive development (see Figure 6.1). As a result, outcome after child TBI is highly variable and often unpredictable, and known adult brain–behavior relationships rarely apply. Further, because of the varied nature (e.g., hematoma, hemorrhage, edema, atrophy) and distribution (e.g., focal, diffuse, multifocal, unilateral, bilateral, cortical, subcortical) of traumatic brain lesions,

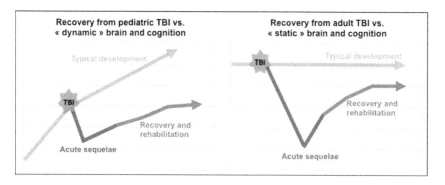

FIGURE 6.1

variability in outcome occurs not only within individuals for specific cognitive processes, but also between individuals of the same age, and within injury severity groups. Given the uneven progress of normal cerebral and cognitive development (Casey, Giedd, & Thomas, 2000; Giedd, Blumenthal, Jeffries, Castellanos, et al., 1999), the range of performance considered to be age-appropriate in children is wide. In those with TBI, poor performance on neuropsychological tests may reflect a developmental delay in acquiring a particular skill or may be a marker of a more serious deficit resulting from disruption of cerebral functioning. Neuropsychological assessment must take into account this variability by ensuring that tests are developmentally appropriate and that test selection is tailored to the individual and hypothesis-driven.

Another important distinction between adult and child neuropsychological assessment concerns the role of parents and other caregivers in the evaluation process. Children are typically in close and constant contact with parents and other adult caregivers who have the ability to provide information on children's functioning, sometimes in domains that are difficult to test directly. These adults can influence children's behavior and the course of their development, and, as such, their perspective and influence on outcome is important to consider. Neuropsychologists can take advantage of access to parents and teachers by soliciting them for information on children's functioning in home, school, extracurricular, and family contexts. This can be particularly useful for domains of functioning that are difficult to evaluate directly in office or hospital settings (e.g., behavior, social relationships, emotions, and physical symptoms in the preverbal child). A neuropsychologist or psychologist may additionally choose to evaluate the impact of parenting style or other parent characteristics (e.g., parental stress, family functioning) on the child. The impact and influence of adult figures naturally differs depending on the period of development (infant, toddler, preschool, childhood, adolescence) and requires appropriate adjustment on the part of the neuropsychologist. This adult-child distinction is particularly relevant in the context of child TBI, as research studies indicate that a number of factors external to the child—such as socio-economic status, family environment, and access to resources and support—have a significant impact on recovery and rehabilitation after brain injury (Taylor, Yeates, Wade, Drotar, et al., 2001; Yeates et al., 1997; Yeates, Taylor, Walz, Stancin, & Wade, 2010).

Goals and Settings

The goal of neuropsychological assessments in children with TBI is framed by the general purposes of pediatric neuropsychological evaluation, which are to 1) provide information regarding the integrity of the brain via comprehensive assessment of its functions; 2) detect and diagnose the presence of symptoms, syndromes, or disorders; 3) gain a better understanding of a child's strengths and weaknesses; 4) orient children toward appropriate rehabilitation, intervention, or support resources based on ability/disability profiles; and 5) monitor change (recovery or deterioration) in performance and evaluate the impact of treatment and interventions. The specific goal of assessment post-TBI is often dependent on the setting in which the neuropsychologist is asked to evaluate the child.

Neuropsychologists are present at most post-injury stages of recovery, though their role differs considerably in first-line and tertiary settings. In acute hospital settings, neuropsychologists usually begin contact with a patient once the child is medically stable (e.g., not in the intensive care unit). At this stage, assessments are brief, basic, conducted at the bedside, and mainly aimed at determining the child's level of consciousness, alertness, and orientation. This may include an assessment of duration of post-traumatic amnesia using standardized measures, such as the Children's Orientation and Amnesia Test (COAT; Ewing-Cobbs, Levin, Fletcher, Miner, & Eisenberg, 1990) or the Westmead Post-Traumatic Amnesia Scale (Marosszeky, Batchelor, Shores, Marosszeky, et al., 1993), though the use of these measures is limited by the child's ability to give a reliable verbal response. Impaired alertness or orientation invalidates other forms of assessment and precludes the possibility of more in-depth neuropsychological testing. If the child has sustained a mild TBI or concussive injury, acute assessments are commonly restricted to documentation and monitoring of post-concussive symptoms (e.g., fatigue, headache, orientation, concentration) via parent or self-report questionnaires, such as the Health and Behavior Inventory (Ayr, Yeates, Taylor, & Brown, 2009) and the Post-Concussive Symptoms Inventory (Gioia, Schneider, Vaughn, & Isquith, 2009).

This initial stage of cognitive assessment might also be performed by a nurse or member of the allied health team (e.g., occupational therapist). Depending on the severity of the injury, monitoring of post-traumatic amnesia may occur over several days or weeks until the child's mental state improves and further neuropsychological investigations are possible.

The goal of the neuropsychological assessment is to gain an overview of affected cognitive systems by screening for possible difficulties and to use this information to make recommendations for further care and follow-up. Questions addressed by the neuropsychologist at that stage could include the following: Should the child be transferred to a rehabilitation unit or center? Can the child be taken home and/or return to school? Is outpatient follow-up necessary? Should the child be assessed again before discharge?

The cursory neuropsychological assessment typical of acute medical settings contrasts with the more in-depth evaluation that occurs in tertiary settings, such as rehabilitation centers, outpatient clinics, school, or private practice, which are conducted under circumstances more conducive to lengthier, targeted assessment. During these assessments, it is typical to obtain information on all spheres of functioning via both standardized and qualitative assessments, in order to produce a complete neurocognitive and behavioral profile, and to make detailed recommendations for improvement of function.

Approach and Methods

An individualized, process-oriented approach is recommended for pediatric neuropsychological assessment, with the clinician selecting tests to administer on the basis of specific diagnostic questions or questions and hypotheses ensuing from acute cognitive screening or a preliminary assessment of intellectual function. This allows the neuropsychologist to take into account the natural variability in cognitive development that exists between children, as well as the unpredictability of outcome after TBI. The use of a fixed battery of tests is rarely appropriate in clinical settings because of lack of flexibility, length of administration, and the danger that important aspects of functioning may be overlooked. An exception to this occurs in the context of sports concussion, where a standard protocol or battery of tests (usually computerized) is often used to serially assess the child or adolescent. This allows the clinician to methodically and precisely document change in performance over time and to make recommendations regarding return to play or to school. Examples of computerized tools used for these purposes are the Immediate Post-Concussion Assessment and Cognitive Testing (ImPACT; (Lovell, Collins, Podell, Powell, & Maroon, 2000), the Computerized Cognitive Assessment Tool (CCAT), CogSport for Kids Signs (Collie, Maruff, Makdissi, McCrory, et al., 2003), and CNS Vital (Gualtieri & Johnson, 2006). However, fixed batteries or lists of tests are also useful, and even essential, in research settings, where the consequences of TBI need to be documented systematically for all patient participants.

Choice of methodology and testing measures is determined by a number of factors. First, fatigue and attention levels will constrain the length and frequency of evaluations in children with TBI. Fatigue, decreased attention and concentration, and persistent headaches are common symptoms of TBI, and the presence and severity of these symptoms will determine how long the neuropsychologist can work with the child, how many breaks are provided, and how often evaluation sessions are scheduled. Patients with severe fatigue or attentional impairments are likely to be too distractible or uncomfortable to provide valid responses to lengthy questions and test items. When the window of opportunity for neuropsychological testing is limited (e.g., a patient is going to be discharged or transferred to another center), the examiner may have to set priorities in the process of testing to obtain the most valuable information.

Second, TBI can cause physical impairments or may occur in concert with other bodily injuries, for which special testing accommodations may have to be made. Serious motor vehicle accidents can cause polytrauma, including severe TBI, orthopedic, pulmonary, and cardiac injuries. In addition, disruption of the brain's motor system can result in partial paralysis, such as hemiplegia, making paper-and-pencil testing that requires a motor response difficult or impossible. Motor impairments can also affect the quality of speech through dysarthria. In these cases, the examiner may need to rely exclusively on verbal or nonverbal responses to acquire valid data. Sensory systems may also be affected and may limit the types of tests used. For example, neurological symptoms in the initial stages post-injury may include blurred or double vision (diplopia), tinnitus (ringing or buzzing in the ears), and hearing loss.

Third, as with neuropsychological assessment in other populations, the age of the child determines what tests are reliable and valid. Traditionally, pediatric measures were derived from validated adult measures; however, with recognition that adult brain-behavior relationships do not always apply to children and that pediatric neuropsychological methods should be distinct and developmentally appropriate, there now exists a wide range of age-appropriate, standardized, normative tests for children and adolescents. Test batteries focusing on specific cognitive functions and individual tools now exist even for the preschool age range (e.g., Korkman, Kirk, & Kemp, 2007; Test of Everyday Attention for Children–A) (Manly, Robertson, Anderson, & Crawford, in press). At the youngest ages (infant, toddler), standardized assessment is possible for global cognitive, language, and motor function via the Bayley Scales of Infant Development (Bayley, 2005). Standardized tools are still lacking for specific cognitive functions at the youngest age ranges.

Fourth, the examiner should gather information from a number of sources, using mixed methodologies. Though the core of neuropsychological assessment relies on standardized testing and comparison to age-normed reference groups, complementary sources of information should be considered. This is especially true after TBI, when behavior and abilities may fluctuate temporally and contextually. For example, a child with TBI may perform adequately on a test of attention in the context of a quiet office space but may be subject to distraction or hypersensitivity to noise and light in a busy classroom. In fact, it is often not until children return to school that the full extent of the impact of TBI can be appreciated and that their responses to environmental demands can be evaluated. A number of parent and caregiver report questionnaires provide ways to quantitatively document cognitive functioning in other contexts (e.g., Conners Parent Rating Scale, Behavior Rating Inventory of Executive Function) (Conners, Sitarenios, Parker, & Epstein, 1998; Gioia & Isquith, 2004; Gioia, Isquith, Guy, & Kenworthy, 2000), and the neuropsychologist should use them to accompany direct quantitative testing and qualitative observations.

Fifth, neuropsychological assessments in children with TBI may need to be more dynamic and occur repeatedly. In light of their ongoing cerebral and cognitive development, children with damage to a particular region of the brain may not show evidence of impairment until a particular developmental skill is expected to emerge or until cognitive demands on the affected system increase. Thus, a child may appear to have intact functioning in a particular domain at early post-injury time points but perform more poorly on the same functions at a follow-up assessment. This underscores the importance of repeated assessments to monitor the progression of function and behavior at multiple post-injury stages and as environmental demands fluctuate (e.g., transition from elementary to high school or from adolescence to adulthood). Evidence from longitudinal follow-up in research settings indicates that some deficits may persist over the very long term or may fluctuate, affecting other functions in the long term (e.g., Anderson, Brown, Newitt, & Hoile, 2011; Anderson, Catroppa, Morse, Haritou, & Rosenfeld, 2000; Catroppa & Anderson, 1999b).

Domains and Tools

Brief, or screening, assessments are typical of the acute and inpatient hospital setting or for mild TBI and concussive injuries and contribute significantly to the identification of children at risk for demonstrating later neuropsychological and functional impairments. However, for a complete picture of a child's functioning following a serious TBI, in-depth assessment of a variety of domains is usually required (once the child is able to manage more challenging testing situations) (see Figure 6.2). A wide variety of standardized measures and tools is available for this purpose and can be chosen with some degree of flexibility according to examiners' preferences and the specific aims of their assessment. The psychometric properties and value of these tools are described in detail in existing references for pediatric neuropsychological assessment, and these works can provide guidance in choosing the best available measures according to the aims of the assessment, domains to be tested, and age of the child (e.g., Baron, 2004; Lezak, 1995).

A complete neuropsychological assessment should target core domains of cognitive functioning within a developmental framework, as well as collect information on peripheral or environmental influences on these domains. Neuropsychological assessment of the full impact of TBI on development should include evaluation or consideration of the following domains.

History, Family, and Pre-Morbid Functioning

History taking is an essential part of the neuropsychological process, because of the influence of developmental information on the interpretation of actual test performance. In the context of child TBI, documentation of **pre-morbid** functioning is of critical importance. Though this is an inexact procedure due to parental bias related to the state of the child following the injury, examiners should gather information on pre-injury function in order to determine as accurately as possible which impairments can be related directly to TBI versus those that may have been present prior to injury. A child who obtains a low average score on a test of intellectual functioning after sustaining TBI may be seen as having an injury-related impairment if he or she was a top student prior to the accident. On the other hand, the same score may be considered normal for a child who struggled academically prior to the injury. In addition, some conditions may be typically present in children who sustain TBI and may or may not worsen after the injury. Studies

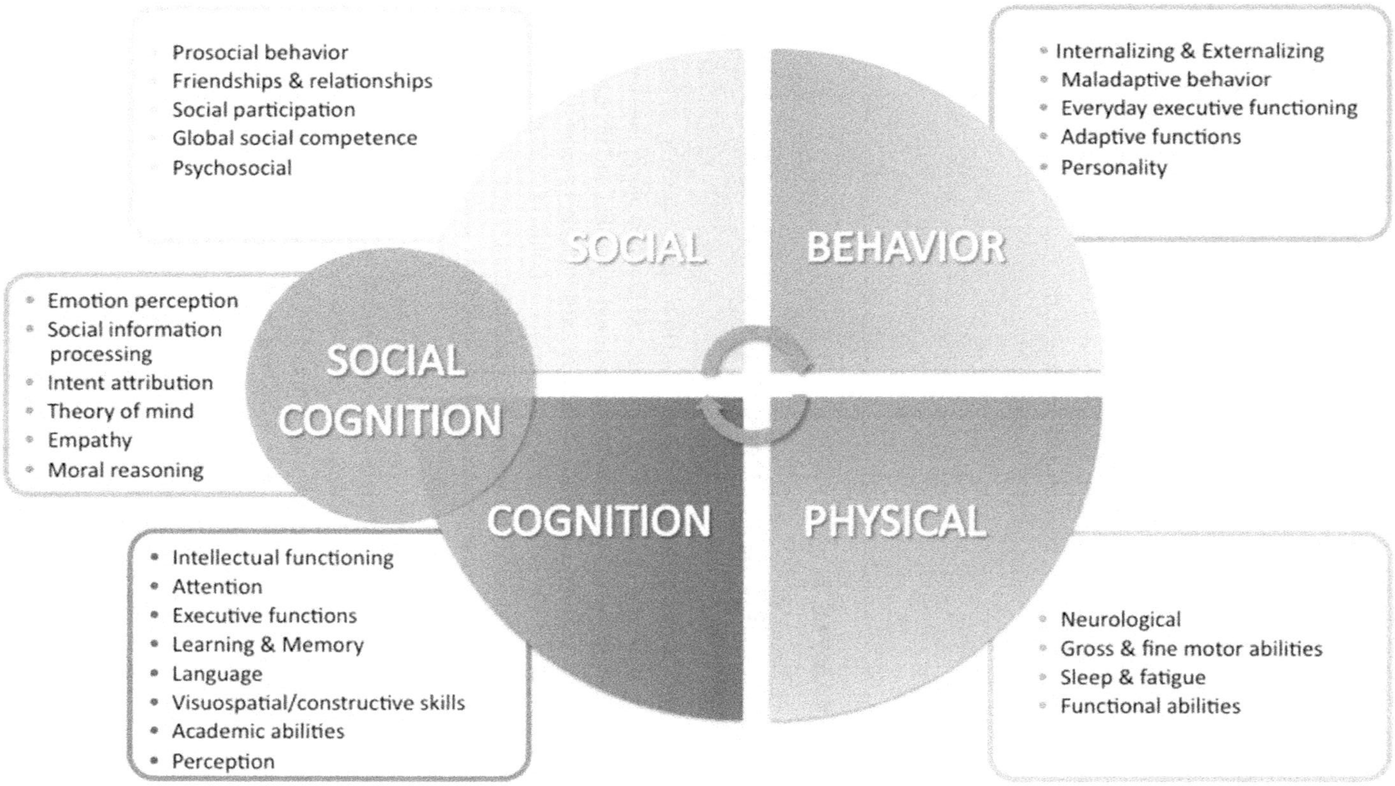

BEHAVIOR
- Internalizing & Externalizing
- Maladaptive behavior
- Everyday executive functioning
- Adaptive functions
- Personality

PHYSICAL
- Neurological
- Gross & fine motor abilities
- Sleep & fatigue
- Functional abilities

SOCIAL
- Prosocial behavior
- Friendships & relationships
- Social participation
- Global social competence
- Psychosocial

SOCIAL COGNITION
- Emotion perception
- Social information processing
- Intent attribution
- Theory of mind
- Empathy
- Moral reasoning

COGNITION
- Intellectual functioning
- Attention
- Executive functions
- Learning & Memory
- Language
- Visuospatial/constructive skills
- Academic abilities
- Perception

FIGURE 6.2

show, for example, that some children who sustain TBI have a history of attention-deficit/hyperactivity disorder (ADHD) (Levin, Hanten, Max, Li, et al., 2007). These children would be expected to exhibit attentional difficulties regardless of the impact of TBI. Information on development and premorbid functioning can be collected via developmental and medical history questionnaires, school report cards, parent questionnaires pertaining to child behavior or other skills, previous assessment and consultation reports, and a detailed parent/child intake interview. The intake interview is an opportunity to gather information pertaining to the child's environment and to family functioning both pre- and post-injury, as these external factors are known to affect children's functioning after TBI. In addition, questionnaires designed to describe and document the impact of the injury on parent and family functioning can be helpful.

CASE EXAMPLE 1

Tim, Differentiating Pre-Injury Characteristics and TBI Symptoms

Injury history. Tim is a 5-year-old boy, admitted to hospital following an accident in which he was knocked from his bike and dragged along the road. He suffered multiple trauma, including a fractured right tibia and fibia, and facial abrasions requiring grafting. Medical records indicated a brief loss of consciousness at the accident scene, and Tim was described as agitated and crying on presentation to the emergency department some 10 minutes later. CT scan was essentially normal, and no neurologic abnormalities were detected, suggestive of a mild TBI.

Pre-injury history. Tim demonstrated some pre-injury behavioral difficulties, including impulsivity, overactivity, and inattention, and he was noted to have acquired speech and language more slowly than his siblings. His parents were both unemployed at the time of his accident, despite having previously stable employment histories. There were reported marital difficulties, and Tim's siblings also exhibited some behavioral difficulties.

Neuropsychology assessment. On assessment, at four weeks post-injury, Tim presented as an active, friendly boy who participated adequately and was generally able to grasp test instructions. He was impulsive and fidgety, particularly toward the end of test sessions. Qualitatively, Tim's expressive language was immature for his age and sometimes difficult to understand. Testing included intellectual evaluation and assessment of verbal skills, new learning, processing speed, and motor skills. Tim's parents also completed questionnaires rating his current behavior. Results indicated that Tim had inconsistent abilities, with age-appropriate nonverbal skills, including new learning and intact motor skills and processing speed. In contrast, verbal skills were within the "Borderline" range, and he displayed impaired language comprehension, expression, verbal knowledge, and verbal memory. Parent ratings of behavior indicated clinically significant problems in attention and hyperactivity domains.

Formulation. Taken together, these data suggest the most likely cause of Tim's difficulties is a pre-existing developmental delay, impacting language and attention primarily, and possibly exacerbated by recent family psychosocial issues. Tim's intact performances in domains usually thought to be vulnerable to brain injury (processing speed, new learning), as well as the mild nature of injury, do not support his post-injury problems being due to brain injury.

Cognitive Functioning

A comprehensive neuropsychological examination of all cognitive domains is usually necessary following child TBI, because of the unpredictable and diffuse nature of most lesions. Although information on lesion location derived from neuroimaging may guide hypothesis testing over the course of a neuropsychological evaluation, the lack of an exact association between location of injury and outcome in children frequently necessitates a complete assessment of cognitive domains that may be affected. Specific domains of cognitive functioning may be affected by direct injury to the brain—resulting, for example, from a focal brain lesion. However, other domains may be affected indirectly through the disruption of functional networks or through secondary injuries, such as swelling and edema, which are likely to affect the brain more diffusely.

Intellectual function. An overview of cognitive integrity or dysfunction typically begins with assessment of intellectual or global cognitive functioning using standardized test batteries (e.g., Bayley Scales of Infant and Toddler Development, Wechsler Scales of Intelligence, Differential Abilities Scale) (Elliott, 2007; Wechsler, 2002, 2003). Though such measures have generally been considered insensitive to the impact of TBI in adults, they may be more useful in the developing child, who may fail to acquire new knowledge and skills following a TBI. As described in Case 2, below, serial testing using these global cognitive measures may demonstrate a failure to maintain expected developmental gains following the injury. The results obtained on these tests can also serve as a basis for the investigation of more specific cognitive domains and for selecting the tools and measures with which to assess them.

CASE STUDY 2

Mark, Severe TBI with Emerging Cognitive Deficits

Mark was a typically developing toddler when he sustained a severe TBI as a result of falling beneath a tractor at age 3 years. Initially unconscious, he was transferred to hospital via air ambulance. On admission, investigations confirmed bilateral frontal lobe contusions and hemorrhage, requiring surgical intervention. Mark remained unconscious for four weeks and received intensive rehabilitation over the months following the accident.

On discharge, two months after the accident, Mark's residual difficulties included restricted expressive and receptive language, severely limited attention, impaired mobility, significant gross and fine motor problems, and poor impulse control. Six months after the accident, Mark continued to experience difficulties with mobility and coordination. His speech was dysfluent, restricting his capacity for communication. Attention and behavioral problems had emerged as major concerns, and his parents reported significant difficulties managing his behavior. Mark's post-injury IQ scores are illustrated below (age at testing noted in brackets).

	2 months (3.6 yrs)	6 months (4.0 yrs)	2 years (5.6 yrs)	4 years (7.6 yrs)	8 years (11.6 yrs)
Verbal IQ	105	104	93	85	70
Nonverbal IQ	100	98	90	88	77

As these results indicate, Mark exhibited age-expected progress in the first six months, probably reflecting some recovery of function in addition to limited developmental progress. After this, his development (measured by global assessment tools) slowed, with minimal improvement over the following years. By eight years post-injury, Mark was functioning well below age level. These results paralleled his school progress. Mark initially commenced mainstream school at age six, requiring full-time support and a modified educational curriculum. By mid-primary school, Mark's considerable problems became difficult to manage within the normal classroom, and he was transferred to a special school for children with intellectual impairment.

Attention. Attentional functions are vulnerable to brain injury, and all types of attention should be tested, including directed (mental and physical state of readiness to respond to a specific stimulus—e.g., wakefulness), selective (selective bias that facilitates that processing of specific information by inhibiting responses to distracting internal or external stimuli), divided (ability to respond simultaneously to multiple tasks), and sustained (capacity to maintain a pattern of responses in a continuous manner, often measured as the fluctuation of performance over time— e.g., fatigue, concentration) forms of attention in both visual and auditory modalities. Working memory (the ability to manipulate and maintain information over the short term) should also be included in the assessment of attentional functions.

Learning and memory. True amnestic disorders are uncommon in the long term after child TBI; however, anterograde and retrograde amnesia may be present in the acute stages post-injury, in addition to amnesia for the event that caused the TBI. Learning and memory functions can be disrupted indirectly due to attentional and executive deficits. Typically, multiple aspects of declarative memory (the capacity to encode and store information in short- and long-term memory and to protect the information from interference) are assessed according to modality (visual and auditory), with consideration of recall interval (immediate, delayed, remote memory) and stage (encoding, consolidation, storage, retrieval). In cases in which the hippocampi may have been directly affected by the injury, it may be useful to differentiate between the integrity of declarative memory (usually associated with the intact functioning of that region) and procedural memory (associated with the integrity of cortico-striatal connections). Prospective memory, which is associated with remembering to perform an action in the future, may be important to consider, especially in cases in which damage to the frontal lobes may also affect executive functions.

Executive function. Executive functioning incorporates a wide range of skills that are central to appropriate daily living, coping, behavior, social, and academic skills and are regulated in large part by the frontal areas of the brain. These skills therefore need to be critically examined following child TBI, with attention to multiple components, including planning (ability to anticipate future events, formulate goals and objectives, put into action a sequence of steps to reach a goal), organization (capacity to coordinate a sequence of steps in a logical, systematic, and strategic manner), inhibition (delay of gratification, self-regulation, self-control), mental flexibility (capacity to alternate between two tasks, incorporate feedback and learn from one's errors, and process information from multiple sources), and abstract reasoning (capacity to analyze information and solve complex problems).

Language. Various aspects of language may be differentially affected by child TBI, and qualitative features of language production and comprehension may be noted from engaging children in conversation during initial stages of the evaluation. Quantitative documentation of specific components of language deserves consideration, including expressive and receptive language components in both written and oral modalities (transmission and comprehension of spoken, symbolic, and written language). Comprehensive assessment should also consider specific subcomponents, such as verbal fluency, phonological processing, comprehension, repetition, expressive and receptive vocabulary, reading, spelling, and writing, as well as more general skills related to conversation and communication (the ability to transmit a message using well-chosen language and appropriate tone of voice, including use of emotional markers, prosody, pragmatics, and nonverbal language). The detection of a language impairment may necessitate referral to a speech therapist for further assessment and intervention. Language abilities should also be differentiated from speech, which refers to the motoric components of language and needs to be assessed by a speech therapist if dysarrthria or other motor production problems are suspected.

Motor, perceptual, and sensory skills. The assessment of perceptual and sensory abilities is sometimes neglected in neuropsychological assessment or may be covered by initial neurological examinations, including tests for extinction, discrimination, perception of dimensions, color, or shapes, and tactile object recognition. Yet, screening for impairments in these areas may be useful, particularly at early stages post-injury, in order to determine whether basic functions have been disrupted by TBI before more complex, higher-order cognitive functions, which often rely on the integrity of sensory and perceptual systems, are assessed. Motor assessment should include screening of both gross and fine motor skills, as well as coordination between left and right hands, integration of motor actions with visual and perceptual skills (visuomotor integration), and both speed and precision of actions. Evaluation of praxis should also be included, to detect presence of any type of apraxia (an inability to perform skilled movements that is not due to a specific physical weakness or loss of sensation). Identification of motor impairments during neuropsychological screening may require referral to a physical therapist and/or occupational therapist for further assessment and intervention.

Visuoperceptive, visuospatial, and visuoconstructive abilities. As with motor, perceptual, and sensory skills, it is important for the neuropsychologist to detect difficulties in visuoperceptive, visuospatial, or visuoconstructive abilities that may affect higher-order functions, such as logical or abstract reasoning. Assessment of skills in this domain includes face/object recognition, visual closure and matching, figure-ground discrimination, visuospatial orientation and integration, mental rotation, and visuomotor construction.

Behavioral and Adaptive Function

Evaluation of behavioral and adaptive functions is an implicit part of the neuropsychological assessment after child TBI. Deviations in behavior are observable qualitatively throughout evaluation sessions; however, accurate assessment of this domain often requires collection of information via third-party sources, because the controlled environment in which neuropsychological testing typically occurs limits the observation of more naturalistic behaviors. There exist a number of standardized questionnaires, which can be useful in gathering information on behavioral, psychosocial, and adaptive skills from parents and teachers, such as the Vineland Adaptive Behavior Scale (Sparrow, Balla, & Cicchetti, 1984), Adaptive

Behavior Assessment System (Harrison & Oakland, 2003), Child Behavior Checklist (Achenbach, Thomas, & Rescorla, 2001), Behavior Assessment System for Children (Reynolds & Kamphaus, 1992), and Strength and Difficulties Questionnaire (Goodman, 1997). Though these are subject to bias from the person completing the questionnaire, they can be helpful to corroborate clinical observations and provide insight into functioning in environments outside the clinic or hospital. Suspected difficulties in behavioral domains may also fall under the responsibility of clinical psychologists or psychiatrists, who can use projective, observational, and therapeutic techniques to gain a better understanding of the difficulties experienced by the child with TBI and to intervene adequately. This is particularly the case where mood disturbance (e.g., depression, anxiety, post-traumatic stress disorder) may have occurred following TBI, requiring long-term follow-up.

Social Cognition and Social Skills

It is now recognized that TBI sustained in childhood may adversely affect social functioning, both through more global adaptive and behavioral dysfunction (Yeates, Bigler, Dennis, Gerhardt, et al., 2007) and through specific socio-cognitive impairments (e.g., Muscara, Catroppa, & Anderson, 2008b; Walz, Yeates, Taylor, Stancin, & Wade, 2010; Wood & Williams, 2008). General outcome measures, for instance—those that provide a rating of adaptive, social, and behavioral functioning—may be helpful in gaining a broad sense of the type of social difficulties that are of concern to parents after their child sustains a TBI (see Muscara & Crowe, 2012, for a review). However, it is also necessary to determine what specific domains of socio-cognitive functioning may be affected, including face and emotion processing, theory of mind and intent attribution, empathy, social information processing and problem solving, and moral reasoning. Though there are a great number of valid experimental tests of social functioning, there are few reliable, standardized tools with which to assess socio-emotional and socio-cognitive function in the field of developmental neuropsychology. The second edition of the NEPSY test battery (Korkman, Kirk, & Kemp, 2007) includes a social perception category, the addition of which reflects a growing recognition that measures of socio-cognitive processes need to be addressed in neuropsychological testing. The development of standardized social evaluation measures is an active area of research and development and is likely to produce a number of interesting assessment options in coming years (see Bruneau-Bhérer, Achim, & Jackson, 2012, for a review of measures).

Academic and Vocational Achievement

Subsequent to disruption of cognitive functions, children with TBI may show difficulties in academic domains, such as language, reading, writing, spelling, and arithmetic (Catroppa, Anderson, Muscara, Morse, et al., 2009; Ewing-Cobbs, Prasad, Kramer, Cox, et al., 2006). These difficulties may become apparent only when the child reintegrates into the school setting. Neuropsychological assessment should consider the impact of injury on these domains both prior to return to school and in the long term to facilitate school reintegration and to provide guidance to colleagues in the school setting concerning avenues for classroom intervention and individualized learning plans to compensate for possible deficits. The Wechsler Individual Achievement Test (Wechsler, 2005) is useful for gaining a broad picture of a child's reading and written language skills, as well as mathematical abilities. Other, more specific, academic tests and tools for diagnosing learning disabilities may then be chosen according to the child's overall academic profile.

Neuropsychological Assessment Domains in Research Settings

Neuropsychological assessment in child TBI research settings has not traditionally followed clear or common guidelines, the particular domains and tools used for testing being driven by specific research questions and hypotheses. However, recent efforts to improve the comparability, comprehensiveness, and scientific rigor of results from clinical TBI trials has brought about the elaboration of guidelines for common measures to be streamlined across studies pertaining to TBI. The recommendations of the National Institute of Neurological Disorders and Stroke (NINDS) for tools and measures (or "Common Data Elements") to be used for TBI research can be consulted online (http://www.commondataelements.ninds. nih.gov/TBI.aspx).

Assessment in Other Domains of Functioning

The evaluation of sequelae and functioning in children with TBI requires the coordination and integration of multiple health professionals from all levels of post-injury services. Members of allied health and rehabilitation disciplines work closely with acute medical care professionals and neuropsychologists and often have a dual role in both assessment and rehabilitation of function. Specific problems detected in early stages of recovery are usually communicated to experts on multidisciplinary teams, enabling a comprehensive and highly specialized approach to the identification and rehabilitation of impairments. Initial clinical assessment is usually followed by referral to members of a rehabilitation team, who conduct further evaluations and identify goals and plans for intervention and recovery.

Occupational Therapy

Occupational therapists are involved in the assessment of children with TBI at different stages of recovery and rehabilitation. Initially, they may play a role in the assessment and monitoring of proper positioning of comatose patients. They also play a role in the global assessment of functional outcomes, especially as they relate to activities of daily living and self-care, such as dressing, eating, hygiene and grooming, safety, transportation, and, in older patients, managing money and making purchases. Such assessments occur directly with the patient, as well as through standardized tools, such as the Pediatric Evaluation of Disability Inventory (Haley, Coster, Ludlow, Haltiwanger, & Andrellos, 1999) and Functional Independence Measure for Children (WeeFIM; Msall, Di Gaudio, Rogers, La Forest, et al., 1994). Assessment of function by occupational therapists also includes social and leisure activities, such as determining a child's preferred activities, areas of interests, hobbies, and social participation (e.g., Children's Assessment of Participation and Enjoyment (CAPE; King, Law, King, Hurley, et al., 2006); Child and Adolescent Scale of Participation (CASP; Bedell, 2009)). Assessment of function extends to the school/work, home, and community environments to determine a patient's level of productivity and to establish how these environments contribute to the patient's overall function (or dysfunction), what resources are available, and what adaptations may be helpful (e.g., to make the home environment safer or more manageable). The work of the occupational therapist occurs in collaboration with members of the medical and rehabilitation team. In particular, occupational therapists may be involved in the assessment of motor function and in determining how motor disability affects activities of daily living, play, writing skills, computer use, and other activities requiring motor coordination. Assessment of motor function includes the evaluation of the child's need for specialized equipment (e.g., wheelchair, splints, communication aids).

Physical Therapy

Physical therapists play a role in the treatment of motor disabilities after TBI. As such, they are initially involved in the assessment of motor functioning after TBI, and they evaluate pain, strength, range of motion, and endurance. Initial assessment involves subjective examination and gathering of information pertaining to the mechanism of injury, history of previous injuries, and type and intensity of pain. Objective assessment includes evaluation of the integrity of all motor systems and determination of short- and long-term goals, leading to the elaboration of a rehabilitation treatment plan (e.g., Gross Motor Function Measure; Linder-Lucht, Verena Othmer, Walther, Vry, et al., 2007). Physical therapists evaluate posture, movement patterns, swelling, deformity, and physical asymmetry.

Speech Therapy and Audiology

Speech and language pathologists (SLPs) are involved in the screening and comprehensive assessment of speech and communication disorders following TBI. Like neuropsychologists, they rely on the use of both standardized (norm-referenced measures) and non-standardized (e.g., observation, interviews) methods to evaluate oral-motor function, speech production, expressive and comprehensive language skills (oral and written), and communication (including social communication and some cognitive aspects related to communication). SLPs also play a role in the assessment of swallowing impairments. TBI can cause difficulties in children's ability to swallow, a problem known as dysphagia. In addition to affecting nutritional intake, dysphagia can result in serious medical problems, such as aspiration and airway obstruction. The *Preferred Practice Patterns for the Profession of Speech-Language Pathology* guidelines, published by the American Speech-Language-Hearing Association (2004), contain a detailed explanation of the assessment procedures recommended for the evaluation of each of the domains listed above. In some cases, speech and language impairments may be related to auditory processing difficulties subsequent to TBI, requiring an audiology assessment. Tinnitus is a frequent consequence of mild TBI, but more serious, long-term auditory processing difficulties require comprehensive assessment including audiometry, testing of acoustic reflexes, typanometry, and testing of the integrity of the central auditory nervous system—for example, using auditory evoked potentials.

Psychology and Neuropsychiatry

Certain mood and personality changes resulting from TBI may require referral and assessment by a pediatric psychologist and/or neuropsychiatrist. Psychologists are instrumental in assessing, characterizing, and providing therapy for mood disorders commonly associated with pediatric TBI (e.g., anxiety, depression), as well as in providing support for psychosocial and academic reintegration in collaboration with social workers and special educators.

In their assessment, neuropsychiatrists emphasize the phenomenology of behavioral disorders after TBI and how these correlate with neurological dysfunction. This may include a diagnostic interview process, review of pre-injury and developmental information, and examination of mental status. Neuropsychiatrists may especially be involved in the evaluation of personality changes (e.g., Adolescent Minnesota Multiphasic Personality Inventory (Graham, Archer, Tellegen, Ben-Porath, & Kaemmer, 2009); Personality Inventory for Children (Lachar, 1992)), psychopathological symptomatology (e.g., Symptom Checklist–Revised) (Derogatos, 1994), and the presence of emotional and mood disturbances after child TBI, such as depression, anxiety, and post-traumatic stress disorder. Gaining a comprehensive picture of the patient's behavioral profile may take several sessions. As medical practitioners, neuropsychiatrists may also integrate their assessment results with those of neurological assessments, such as neuroimaging and electrophysiological scanning, laboratory tests (blood, urine), and pharmacological history.

Sleep and Fatigue

The assessment of potential sleep-wake disturbances and fatigue problems after pediatric TBI has emerged as an important domain that requires monitoring over time. Disturbed sleep is one of the most frequently reported post-injury symptoms, even after mild TBI (Hooper, Alexander, Moore, Sasser, et al., 2004). Fatigue has also been described as a common and persistent symptom of pediatric TBI. It can accompany sleep-wake disturbances or be observed as an isolated symptom (Limond, Dorris, & McMillan, 2009). Both post-traumatic sleep-wake disturbances and fatigue can compromise the rehabilitation process and return to activities. They can also seriously impact performance in multiple cognitive, physical, social, and functional domains. Because their assessment does not belong to a particular profession, clinicians involved in the continuum of care after pediatric TBI should be aware of the implications of sleep and fatigue problems on other domains of functioning, as well as how to measure sleep quality and fatigue.

A review of methodologies used to assess sleep and fatigue after pediatric TBI indicates that indirect and subjective measures, such as sleep diaries and questionnaires, dominate the empirical literature (Gagner, Landry-Roy, Lainé, & Beauchamp, 2015) and are also used in some clinical settings. Questionnaires used to assess sleep are varied, though the most commonly used is the Children's Sleep Habits Questionnaire (Owens, Spirito, & McGuinn, 2000). The Child Behavior Checklist (Achenbach & Edelbrock, 1991), which includes a sleep subscale, and the Epworth Sleepiness Scale (King, Crawford, Wenden, Moss, & Wade, 1995) are examples of other questionnaires that are used to assess sleep. The Pediatric Quality of Life Inventory Multidimensional Fatigue Scale (PedsQL MFS; Varni, Burwinkle, Katz, Meeske, & Dickinson, 2002; Varni, Burwinkle, & Szer, 2004) is the most frequently used questionnaire to document fatigue in children with brain injury (Crichton, Knight, Oakley, Babl, & Anderson, 2015). Questionnaires targeting broader post-concussive symptoms can also be used to screen for fatigue and/or sleep-wake disturbances; however, the questions included are generally imprecise, making it difficult to determine what types of problems are experienced.

The use of objective methods such as polysomnography, which is considered the gold standard of sleep assessment methods, is relatively rare in pediatric research settings (Gagner et al., 2015). This is likely to be a function of the more invasive nature of polysomnographic recordings, which make measurement in younger populations more challenging and less feasible. Actigraphy, which uses a device similar to a wristwatch that contains an accelerometer to record movement and determine sleep and wake episodes, may be a useful, objective alternative, but it is limited by the fact that it provides only an indirect measure of sleep. Clinical settings with specialized sleep clinics may provide useful objective and comprehensive assessment of sleep-wake disturbances in controlled environments.

Conclusions

Accurate assessment of the consequences of pediatric TBI is crucial to the appropriate management, follow-up, rehabilitation, and reintegration of young patients, and it requires multi-modal evaluation of a variety of domains of functioning. Comprehensive assessment of outcome calls upon not only extensive neuropsychological and psychological expertise for the identification of potential cognitive, behavioral, academic, adaptive, social, and psychological difficulties, but also multidisciplinary involvement for the diagnosis and detection of possible physical, functional, psychiatric, and language impairments. It is imperative that such assessments take into account the developmental context of brain injuries and that clinicians and researchers bear in mind the psychometric properties as well as the limitations of available assessment tools. Though some areas of functioning have well-established materials and recommendations for standardized and comprehensive assessment (e.g., core cognition, behavior scales), other domains and their related tools are rapidly evolving (e.g., social cognition, computerized testing).

7

OUTCOMES AND PREDICTORS OF CHILD TBI

Introduction

Traumatic brain injury in children has been linked to a range of cognitive and behavioral consequences, in keeping with current knowledge regarding brain-behavior relationships in the developing brain. As described in Chapter 3, closed-head injuries (CHI) in particular are characterized by a typical pattern of brain pathology and functional deficit. Following impact, damage occurs due to the initial compression of the head against an object and the resultant acceleration-deceleration movement of the brain contents inside the skull. These movements can stretch and tear nerve axons and blood vessels, resulting in both focal and diffuse axonal injury (Fennell & Mickle, 1992; Levin & Kraus, 1994). Secondary effects may also occur, including hypoxia, seizures, edema, disrupted neurochemical processes, and raised intracranial pressure (Amacher, 1988; Fennell & Mickle, 1992; Hynd & Willis, 1988; Yeates, 1999). It is the complexities of these primary and secondary processes that result in brain injuries differing in their level of severity, which variably affect both short- and long-term outcome in cognitive, social, behavioral, and functional areas, suggesting that TBI should be defined and managed as a chronic process (Masel & DeWitt, 2010). Therefore, the aim of this chapter is to provide an overview of (a) outcomes for mild, moderate, and severe injury in the acute/post-acute phase and in the longer term and (b) predictors of outcome in both acute/post-acute and longer-term post-injury.

Outcome Following Concussion and Mild TBI

Acute/Post-Acute Outcomes

As noted in Chapter 2, mild TBI and concussion (referred to as mTBI) constitute 90% of all child TBI (Crowe et al., 2009; Kraus, Fife, Cox, Ramstein, & Conroy,

1986; Langlois et al., 2006; Russo, Rice, Chern, & Raftos, 2012; Valerio & Illes, 2011; Yeates, 2010), and is most prevalent between the ages of 5 and 14 (Asarnow et al., 1995). Common causes include sporting injuries and falls (Andersson, Sejdhage, & Wage, 2012; Browne & Lam, 2005). Understanding the epidemiology of mTBI is difficult, as the criteria that define a mTBI may be variable (Tellier, Marshall, Wilson, Smith, et al., 2009), injuries often go unrecognized or unreported, and, of those who seek medical attention, many are not followed up or are lost to follow-up. Methodologies, assessment tools, and imaging protocols between studies are also diverse, leading to variability and inconsistencies in findings following an mTBI (Carroll, Cassidy, Holm, Kraus & Coronado, 2004; Elson & Ward, 1994; Evans, 1992; Mayer, Ling, Yang, Pena, et al., 2012; McDonald, Saykin, & McAllister, 2012; McKinlay, 2009; Shenton, Hamoda, Schneiderman, Bouix, et al., 2012). Some argue that these mild insults are associated with either no detectable sequelae or full recovery (Asarnow et al., 1995; Babikian, Satz, Zaucha, Light, et al., 2011, Babikian, McArthur, & Asarnow, 2012; Ettenhofer & Abeles, 2009; Levin et al., 1987, Maillard-Wermelinger, Yeates, Taylor, Rusin, et al., 2009; Papero, Prigatano, Snyder, & Johnson, 1993; Ponsford et al., 1999), while others report significant, ongoing problems (Asarnow, Satz, Light Lewis, & Neumann, 1991; Boll, 1983; Clarke, Genat, & Anderson, 2012; Gronwall, Wrightson, & McGinn, 1997; Hamilton & Keller, 2010; Jonsson Elgmark, & Andersson, 2012; Kaldoja & Kolk, 2012; Massagli, Fann, Burington, Jaffe, et al., 2004; McKinlay et al., 2002, 2009; Scherwath, Sommerfeldt, Bindt, Nolte, et al., 2011; Toledo, Lebel, Becerra, Minster, et al., 2012; Yeates et al., 2012).

In the acute phase following mTBI, there is a high risk of post-concussive symptoms, characterized by transient impairments in cognition (memory, attention, executive function, and processing speed), physical function (fatigue, headache, nausea), and psychological status (irritability, mood change, emotional dysregulation). In adults, these symptoms have typically been found to remit in 7–10 days (Broglio & Puetz, 2008; Guskiewicz, Ross, & Marshall, 2001; Iverson et al., 2006, 2012). Recovery timelines are less well defined for children and adolescents, with some suggestion that recovery is more protracted (Choe, Babikian, DiFiori, Hovda, & Giza, 2012; Field, Collins, Lovell, & Maroon, 2003; McCrory, Collie, & Anderson, 2004; Purcell, 2009). Supporting this view, a recent study by Barlow and colleagues (2010) found an elevated risk of post-concussional symptoms in children and adolescents with mTBI to at least three months post-injury. Taylor and colleagues (Taylor, Dietrich, Nuss, Wright, et al., 2010; Yeates, Taylor, Rusin, Bangert, et al., 2009) have extended these findings and note that post-concussional symptoms reflecting more cognitive problems (e.g., reduced attention) are persistent and that children with persisting symptoms are more likely to demonstrate abnormalities on high-resolution neuroimaging.

This delayed recovery pattern in children and adolescents post-mTBI, though not yet well understood, is argued to affect about 20% of all victims. Some potential explanations are individual differences in the physiological response to mechanical stress. Furthermore, the geometry of the child's skull and brain mean that a 100%

to 200% greater impact force is required to produce the same clinical symptoms in children as adults. Similarly, the head, relative to body size, is disproportionately larger in the child and also less stable. The immature skull is more flexible than the adult skull, leading to a greater preponderance of diffuse injury, and less focal injury, in children. In addition, the greater muscle mass of adults, especially in athletes, means that the force of impact is diluted through the upper torso rather than being concentrated in the head as it is with younger athletes (Field et al., 2003; Ommaya, Goldsmith, & Thibault, 2002).

Delayed Recovery, Longer-Term Outcome, and Recovery from mTBI

Characteristic sequelae of mTBI and concussion in children and adolescents include reduced attention, slowed response speeds, memory impairment, fatigue, and irritability (Anderson et al., 2001; McCrory et al., 2013), skills that are pivotal for day-to-day activities such as acquiring new knowledge and skills and attending to schoolwork. In addition to the cognitive sequelae of concussion, children may also experience post-concussion behavioral difficulties not typically observed in the adult population, including headache or pressure in the head, dizziness, fatigue, sleep disturbance, restlessness, sensitivity to noise and vision, blurred or double vision, nausea, and tinnitus (Taylor et al., 2010; Yeates et al., 2009).

However, controversy exists with regard to the long-term resolution of post-concussion symptoms (Lee, 2007). In a meta-analysis of outcome two years following mTBI in childhood, Babikian and Asarnow (2009) identified few, if any, impairments in intellectual ability, attention, and memory function. However, clinically, it is frequently reported that a subgroup of injured children do not show full resolution of all symptoms and can demonstrate residual psychological (e.g. anxiety, irritability, depression) and cognitive (e.g., reduced speed of information processing and executive control, poor memory and attention) problems. These observations are supported by a number of researchers (Anderson et al., 2001; Catale, Marique, Closser, & Meulemans, 2009; Hessen, Anderson, & Nestvold, 2008; Klonoff & Lamb, 1996; McKinlay et al., 2002, 2009; Miller, 1996; Ponsford et al., 1999; Stablum, Mogentaale, & Umilta, 1996), although it is important to note that such problems may be associated with high risk factors, such as young age at injury, abnormalities on clinical investigation, and pre-injury behavioral or cognitive problems.

In order to explain inconsistencies in findings, mTBI has more recently been divided into mild and mild-complicated categories, the latter characterized by subtle structural brain abnormalities, the possibility of neurochemical effects (Hessen et al., 2008; Roberts, Manshad, Bushnell, & Hines, 1995; Yeates, 1999), and persisting post-concussional symptoms (Dikmen, Machamer, Winn, & Temkin, 1995). Fay and colleagues (2009) investigated a group of children, aged 8–15 years at time of injury, classified as complicated or uncomplicated mild TBI, over a 12-month period. They found that children with a complicated injury and of lower cognitive ability were more vulnerable to cognitive symptoms and high levels of post-concussive symptoms over time. Other predictors of poor neurocognitive outcome following mTBI have included premorbid behavioral and learning problems and low parental education (Babikian, McArthur, & Asarnow, 2012).

As mentioned in previous chapters, though comprehensive neuropsychological evaluation is important in more severe TBI, such approaches are less common following mTBI and concussive injuries. Contemporary approaches to assessment of the consequences of these injuries usually include post-concussion symptom checklists and screening tools, frequently computer-based, that focus on evaluation of key domains, such as attention, executive function, and processing speed, and which can be validly repeated in the weeks and months post-injury, to monitor recovery. Where symptoms persist, full neuropsychological evaluation is commonly pursued (West & Marion, 2014).

Moderate to Severe TBI Outcome

Acute/Post-Acute and Longer-Term Outcomes Following Moderate to Severe TBI

Studies of outcome and recovery from moderate to severe TBI in preschool and school-aged children (refer to Table 7.1) have identified acute and persisting impairments (Babikian & Asarnow, 2009) in a number of cognitive domains, including attention and information processing, memory, and executive function. In the main, these problems reflect damage to brain regions subsuming these skills, specifically anterior brain regions and axonal connections. Behavioral and social disturbances also occur and may be due to underlying brain disruption, pre-injury and environmental risks (pre-injury learning and behavior problems, adjustment difficulties, family burden and stress, social disadvantage), or a combination of all these factors.

Attention and information processing. Attentional impairment and slowed processing speed are the hallmark symptoms of serious TBI and have been found to persist with time, putting the young person at risk in his or her daily environment, where he or she may struggle to acquire new knowledge, complete tasks in a timely manner, and interact appropriately with peers. Current neuroscience models identify several components of attention and information processing that are argued to be subsumed by an integrated neural network, involving frontal, temporal, and parietal brain regions as well as subcortical structures.

Sustained attention, or *vigilance,* refers to the capacity to maintain arousal and alertness over time. Selective attention is the ability to select target information while ignoring irrelevant stimuli and to differentially process simultaneous sources of information. *Shifting attention* and *divided attention* can be viewed as the "executive" aspects of the attention system; they refer to the ability to change attentive

TABLE 7.1 Consequences of Child Traumatic Brain Injury—From Childhood to Adulthood

Domain	Specific skills
Neurological impairment	Gross and fine-motor incoordination
	Cranial nerve function/sensory loss
	Speech—e.g., aphasia
	Medical complications—e.g., epilepsy
Cognitive impairment	Intellectual impairment
	Attention/Speed of processing
	Memory and learning
	Language
	Executive function
Educational impairment	Reduced progress—e.g., reading, arithmetic
	Processing difficulties—e.g., attention, processing speed, memory
	Writing difficulties
	Need for specialist placement or support
Adaptive/Emotional/Behavioral	Adjustment difficulties—e.g., reduced self-esteem
	Psychiatric disorders—e.g., depression, anxiety, post-traumatic stress
	Regulatory dysfunction: disinhibition, impulsivity, apathy, reduced insight
Social consequences	Social withdrawal and isolation
	Social anxiety
	Inappropriate social skills, reduced social awareness
Lifestyle change	Reduced independence
	Impaired functional communication and mobility
	Increased need for additional assistance
	Reduced recreational options
	Difficulties maintaining pre-injury relationships

Source: Adapted from Anderson & Catroppa (2006).

focus in a flexible and adaptive manner and to divide one's attention between two or more competing sources of information, respectively. *Attentional control* includes the ability to monitor and inhibit responses. *Speed of processing* refers to the rate at which activities may be completed and so is often considered to underpin the efficiency of the entire system (Anderson, 2002; Mirsky, Anthony, Duncan, Ahearn, et al., 1991; Posner & Peterson, 1990; Stierwalt & Murray, 2002; Stuss, Shallice, Alexander, & Picton, 1995).

Research investigating attentional and processing skills in a pediatric population is limited, with developmental implications poorly considered (Anderson, 2002; Anderson, Anderson, et al., 2001; Betts, McKay, Maruff, & Anderson, 2006; Kail, 1986; Manly, Anderson, Robertson, & Nimmo-Smith, 1999; McKay,

Halperin, Schwartz, & Sharma, 1994; Rebok, Smith, Pascualvaca, Mirsky, et al., 1997), and contrasting results have been reported. In early cross-sectional studies, Timmermans and Christensen (1991) investigated children with TBI aged 5 to 16 years and found evidence for impairments in sustained attention but not in selective attention. In support of these results, Kaufmann, Fletcher, Levin, Miner, and Ewing-Cobbs (1993) also identified specific deficits in sustained attention in their school-age sample. Others have reported additional attentional weakness following TBI, including selective attention (Dennis, Wilkinson, Koski, & Humphreys, 1995), divided attention (Ginstfeldt & Emanuelson, 2010), speed of processing (Anderson & Pentland, 1998; van Zomeren & Brouwer, 1994), and more global attention deficit profiles (Catroppa & Anderson, 1999a, 2003; Park, Allen, Barney, Ringdahl, & Mayfield, 2009).

In our lab, we have monitored attention and its recovery in a prospective, longitudinal study, involving a series of follow-ups in a group of children sustaining injury between 8–12 years of age. At two years post-injury, using a computer-based continuous performance paradigm, difficulties were evident for children with moderate to severe TBI in both sustained attention and shifting attention, particularly on more complex tasks, with psychomotor slowness also apparent. Steepest recovery was evident for the severe TBI group; however, even two years post-TBI, attention skills were below those of children who had sustained only mild or moderate injuries (Catroppa & Anderson, 2005).

We have also examined attention and processing speed outcomes after injury in early childhood (2–7 years), with a somewhat different pattern of findings. At 30 months post-injury, no impairment of sustained attention was found; however, children with severe TBI presented with reduced selective attention, impaired response inhibition, and slowed processing (Anderson et al., 2005c). At five years post-injury, results revealed that these attention and processing speed deficits persist, particularly following severe TBI. In addition, emerging deficits were apparent in higher-order attention skills (shifting attention, divided attention), suggesting that impairments in specific aspects of attention and information processing may not become apparent until later in childhood, when they would be expected to emerge as part of the normal developmental sequence (Catroppa, Anderson, Morse, Haritou, & Rosenfeld, 2007), with attentional difficulties again noted at 10 years post-injury (Catroppa et al., 2011). Ginstfeldt and Emanuelson (2010) completed an evaluation of the types of deficits evident after pediatric TBI. They concluded that divided and sustained attention are highly sensitive to TBI, with attention span most resistant, and shifting and selective attention in between.

Advances in neuroimaging may also contribute to our understanding of the impact of child TBI on this domain. For example, Kramer and colleagues (2008) examined attentional outcome using a functional MRI paradigm, with a group of children who sustained their injuries in early childhood. These authors reported that though similar brain networks were activated, when compared to a healthy control group, children with TBI demonstrated significantly greater activation in frontal and parietal areas, suggesting they required additional brain resources to perform similarly to controls.

Memory and learning. Memory has been described as an integrated system in which information is registered from the environment, encoded, and stored for later retrieval (e.g., Baddeley, 1990; Cowan, 1995). Most theories argue for a working model (van Zomeren & Brouwer, 1994), in which the memory system can direct attention, implement strategies (e.g., rehearsal), and control retrieval.

Like attention, the memory system is subsumed by a complex neural network, involving limbic structures and anterior brain regions, areas that are vulnerable to the impact of TBI (Beauchamp, Ditchfield, Babl, Kean, et al., 2011; Beauchamp, Catroppa, Godfrey, Morse, et al., 2011). Not surprisingly, then, following child TBI, difficulties are commonly reported in various memory components, including immediate, short-term, delayed, complex multitrial learning (Aaro Jonsson, Smedler, Leis Ljungmark, & Emanuelson, 2009; Catroppa & Anderson, 2002; Farmer, Haut, Williams, Kapila, et al., 1999; Horneman & Emanuelson, 2009; Van Heugten, Hendriksen, Rasquin, Dijcks, et al., 2006; Yeates, Blumenstein, Patterson, & Delis, 1995), working memory (Levin, Hanten, et al., 2004; Mandalis, Kinsella, Ong, & Anderson, 2007), prospective memory (McCauley & Levin, 2004; Ward, Shum, McKinlay, Baker, & Wallace, 2009), and implicit/explicit memory (Lah, Epps, Levick, & Parry, 2011; Ward, Shum, Dick, McKinlay, & Baker-Tweney, 2004; Ward, Shum, Wallace, & Boon, 2002).

Levin and Eisenberg (1979) provided one of the first cross-sectional studies addressing memory impairment following child TBI, documenting deficits in both verbal learning and visual recognition. Later, they extended their work to show that though verbal learning difficulties were present regardless of age at injury, visual recognition problems were greater for younger children. Others have reported a deterioration or failure to keep pace with healthy peers over time post-injury for aspects of memory function (Donders, 1993). These findings emphasize the importance of employing a developmental framework, with skills undergoing development at the time of injury potentially more vulnerable to disruption.

Standard clinical measures, including multitrial learning tasks (e.g., list learning), provide an opportunity to assess multiple aspects of memory and learning—for example, short-term memory, encoding, storage, and retrieval. Studies using such approaches have often identified weaknesses in all aspects of learning for children with severe TBI, regardless of modality (i.e., verbal or visual) (Catroppa & Anderson; 2002, 2007; Farmer et al., 1999, 2002; Lowther & Mayfield, 2004; Wright & Schmitter-Edgecombe, 2011; Yeates et al., 1995). In contrast, mild to moderate injuries are associated with better memory outcomes, with most studies describing few problems in these groups. An exception, however, comes from the work of Yeates et al. (1995), who found that children with mild to moderate injuries showed poorer than expected recall after delay. Longitudinal studies confirm that these memory and learning problems persist for at least two years post-TBI (Catroppa & Anderson, 2002, 2007).

Several studies have administered more experimental memory measures to gain a more fine-grained understanding of memory and learning skills following child TBI. For example, Harris (1996), using an overt rehearsal free recall task, found that children with severe TBI presented with impaired verbal recall; they used simple rehearsal strategies and an inefficient passive rehearsal strategy. Consistent with these findings, Hanten and colleagues (Hanten, Bartha, & Levin, 2000; Hanten, Dennis, Zhang, Barnes, et al., 2004) showed that more severely injured children were less able to modify their rehearsal strategies and were limited in the use of metamemory and metacognitive skills, such as estimation of memory span and judgments of recall. Similarly, Crowther and colleagues (2011) found that in children aged 5–15 years, and at 24 months post-injury, greater injury severity was associated with poorer performance on prospective judgments of memory performance and learning strategies.

Imaging studies have recently explored the neural underpinnings of these memory difficulties. Salorio and colleagues (2005) found that, at one year following childhood injury, frontal and/or temporal lesion volumes were predictive of memory performance. Importantly, lesion volume in extra-fronto-temporal areas was even more significantly predictive of memory outcome. Interpreting their results, these authors suggested that, in more severe injuries, diffuse axonal injury may disrupt the neural circuits involved in memory functions.

Language. Though aphasias are rare following child TBI, clinical reports frequently document impairments in communication, including slowed speech, dysfluency, poor logical sequencing of ideas, and word-finding difficulties (Dennis, 1989). In one of the earliest studies to comprehensively assess language outcomes, Ewing-Cobbs, Levin, Eisenberg, and Fletcher (1987) compared mild and moderate TBI with respect to four aspects of language function—naming, expressive and receptive skills, and writing capacity. They identified a significant dose-response relationship, with severe TBI associated with poor performance on all language tasks. Greatest deficits were evident for writing and expressive skills, and these findings have been consistently replicated (Barca, Cappelli, Amicuzi, Apicella, et al., 2009; Campbell & Dolloghan, 1990; Hallett, 1997).

In our team's prospective longitudinal study (Anderson et al., 1997) we showed that, despite having age-appropriate language skills pre-injury, severely injured children exhibited globally impaired performance on tasks of naming, verbal fluency, storytelling, receptive vocabulary, and verbal comprehension. These difficulties persisted to 12 months post-injury with little evidence of recovery. Children with mild to moderate TBI exhibited no such deficits, either at acute or at 12-month assessments. Ewing-Cobbs and coworkers (Ewing-Cobbs et al., 1987) reported similar findings and also note no recovery in the second year post-injury in language skills. Taken together, these various results suggest that there are some differential residual language deficits evident post-TBI, at least in young children, in keeping with the notion that language skills in this age group are rapidly developing and may be particularly vulnerable to disruption.

Following the direction of adult studies, early work by Jordan, Murdoch, and Buttsworth (1991) investigated pragmatics and higher-order processing skills and indicated that post-TBI children did not perform differently on tasks of spontaneous story production or narrative measures when compared to age-matched controls. These authors highlighted the need to observe discourse in a conversational setting in order to evaluate functional difficulties. Conversely, other studies of narrative discourse have found deficits at least one year post-injury, including disruption in story structure (Chapman, Culhane, Levin, Harward, et al., 1992), dysfluency (Biddle, McCabe, & Bliss, 1996), poor knowledge of ambiguous words in context and limited understanding of metaphoric expressions (Dennis & Barnes, 1990), and difficulties with syntax, semantics, and pragmatics (Didus, Anderson, & Catroppa, 1999; Jordan & Murdoch, 1994, Walz, Yeates, Taylor, Stancin, & Wade, 2011). With such impairments, the use of language for effective social interaction is often compromised, resulting in poor communication, a lack of cohesion in discourse, and difficulties at the level of cognitive organization (Capruso & Levin, 1992, Catroppa & Anderson, 2004; Chapman, Gamino, Cook, Hanten, et al., 2006; Chapman, McKinnon, Levin, Song, et al., 2001; Chapman, Sparks, Levin, Dennis, et al., 2004; Ewing-Cobbs, Brookshire, Scott, & Fletcher, 1998; Ewing-Cobbs, Prasad, Swank, Kramer, et al., 2012; Goldstein & Levin, 1992; Hanten et al., 2004; Marquardt, Stoll, & Sussman, 1988; Sullivan & Riccio, 2010).

In order to explore the impact of TBI on language during the acquisition phase, Morse and colleagues (1999) investigated language skills in children between the ages of 4 and 6 years at injury versus healthy controls. Though standard clinical measures detected no group differences, the results of the discourse analysis revealed a trend for the severe TBI group to use fewer communication units compared to control and mild TBI groups, in keeping with clinical reports of difficulties communicating effectively in everyday situations. Subsequently, Hanten and colleagues identified high-level language problems and verbal dysfluency following child TBI (Hanten, Levin, & Song, 1999).

Vu, Babikian, and Asarnow (2011) conducted a meta-analysis of academic and language function outcomes for children post-TBI. Their main findings indicated that though children with mild TBI exhibited no significant deficits, for those with moderate TBI significant deficits were evident in academic skills. With regard to those with severe injury, deficits were found in all areas, with expressive and receptive skills showing a slower rate of recovery and remaining more impaired than other skills over time.

The neural substrate of language networks and associated language-related behavioral impairments in children post-TBI was investigated by Karunanayaka et al. (2007) using an fMRI paradigm. In studying eight children post-TBI, aged 6–9 years, compared to an orthopedic control group, these researchers found that children post-TBI had significantly different brain activation patterns in language circuitry (perisylvian language area).

Executive functions. Executive functions (EF) have been defined as a set of inter-related skills necessary to maintain an appropriate problem-solving set for attainment of a future goal. EFs are generally agreed to include one or more of the following: (1) attentional control; (2) strategic planning and problem-solving; (3) cognitive flexibility of thought and action; and (4) concept formation/abstraction, and are argued to be subsumed by the prefrontal cortex, which is particularly vulnerable following TBI (Anderson et al., 2001; Lezak, 1993; Stuss & Benson, 1986; Weyandt & Willis, 1994).

Attentional control. Ewing-Cobbs and colleagues (2004) assessed young children injured prior to age 6 with moderate to severe TBI at an average of one or two years post-injury. When compared to a community group, children with TBI performed more poorly on measures of inhibitory control and working memory, skills that undergo rapid development in early childhood and thus may be more vulnerable to disruption. This finding has been supported by a number of other researchers (Conklin, Salorio, & Slomine, 2008, Ewing-Cobbs et al., 2004; Levin et al., 2004; Mandalis et al., 2007; Sinopoli & Dennis, 2012), who also reported working memory and inhibition deficits in children following TBI.

More recent literature has focused on the effect of TBI on self-regulation (e.g., Ganesalingham, Sanson, Anderson, & Yeates, 2006). Ganesalingham and colleagues (2006) investigated a group of children two to five years post-injury and compared them to healthy controls. Results indicated deficits in self-regulation and, further, that the self-regulation domain mediated social and behavioral outcomes (Ganesalingham, Sanson, Anderson, & Yeates, 2007).

Strategic planning and problem-solving. Clinically, poor organization and problem-solving skills are frequently described in survivors of child TBI (Jacobs & Anderson, 2002; Levin, Song, Ewing-Cobbs, & Roberson, 2001; Levin, Song, Scheibel, Fletcher, et al., 1997; Schmidt, Hanten, Xiaodi, Vasquez, et al., 2012); however, until relatively recently, there has been little literature addressing this domain. Aspects of EF, via the use of a multidimensional party-planning task, were examined in a group of adolescents who had sustained TBI during childhood (Pentland, Todd, & Anderson, 1998; Todd, Anderson, & Lawrence, 1996). The party-planning task involved designating a series of tasks to four different people, each within a specific time frame and constrained by certain conditions, in order to ensure a well-organized party. Though adolescents with mild injuries performed similarly to controls, those with moderate to severe TBI were significantly impaired in their capacity to take into account the multiple steps required to complete the tasks, suggesting impairments in monitoring performance, decision making, and capacity to allocate attentional resources effectively (Ornstein, Levin, Chen, Hanten, et al., 2009).

Taking a more ecological perspective, Sesma, Slomine, Ding, and McCarthy (2009) investigated EF in 330 children following mild to severe TBI using a questionnaire-based measure of day-to-day function. In comparison to ortho-pedic controls, the group with TBI performed more poorly at 3 and 12 months post-injury. Similarly, using a naturalistic assessment tool, Chevignard and colleagues (2009) examined the ability of child survivors of TBI to complete a cooking task to assess planning and organizational skills. These authors found that the TBI group performed more poorly than healthy controls when required to be attentive, follow rules, plan, and problem-solve.

Metacognitive skills, including knowledge appraisal and knowledge management, have also been examined following child TBI (Dennis, Barnes, Donnelly, Wilkinson, & Humphreys, 1996). "Appraisal" skills involve fact-based knowledge gained from experience and stored in long-term memory, whereas "management" skills involve maintaining and revising ongoing performance and making judgments where necessary. It was found that children with TBI and younger normally developing children performed poorly in both appraisal and management areas. Furthermore, even with a relevant information base, children with TBI were not always able to engage metacognitive processes. As mentioned in an earlier section, Hanten and colleagues (Hanten, Bartha, & Levin, 2000; Hanten et al. 2004; Hanten, Scheibel, Li, Oomer, et al., 2006) also showed that children post-injury were compromised in the use of metamemory and metacognitive skills and in decision-making skills.

Cognitive flexibility and concept formation/abstraction. In an earlier study (Levin et al., 1997), it was shown that post-injury, children presented with difficulties on tasks requiring the use of concept formation and cognitive flexibility. More recently, Anderson and Catroppa (2005) assessed cognitive flexibility and abstract reasoning skills at two years post-TBI, using a sample of 12-year-old children, in whom it was assumed that executive skills would be quite well developed. Children with severe TBI demonstrated deficits in both cognitive flexibility and abstract reasoning. Similarly, Nadebaum, Anderson, and Catroppa (2007) investigated EF in children injured prior to the age of 12 years, at five years post-injury, and results provided support for the presence of long-term EF deficits in the area of cognitive flexibility. Theory of Mind tasks (e.g., measuring intentions, perspective taking) have shown to discriminate between children post-TBI and control children, thereby demonstrating that early injury can impair these fundamental skills required for everyday communication and function (Dennis, Simic, Taylor, Bigler, et al., 2012; Tonks, Williams, Frampton, Yates, et al., 2007; Turkstra, Williams, Tonks, & Frampton, 2008; Walz et al., 2009, 2010).

Long-term impairments in executive skills following child TBI. Clinical observations of persisting deficits in EF have reported many implications for aspects of daily living. Without efficient EF, not only are impairments seen in areas such as attentional control, planning, flexibility, and organization, but secondary difficulties may arise in social skills and in coping with day-to-day interactions and expectations.

Outcomes greater than five years post-injury, in the area of EF, were investigated by Muscara et al. (2008a). The sample, injured between 8 and 12 years of age, and aged between 16 and 22 years at the time of assessment, were 7–10 years post-injury, and at a time of transition into adulthood. Findings indicated that those with more severe injury displayed a higher degree of executive dysfunction on both standardized and functional assessments. Beauchamp et al. (2011) investigated 40 adolescents at 10 years post-injury and found that compared to a control group, those with severe injuries had poorer performance on goal-setting and processing speed tasks, highlighting the need for ongoing management and support.

As in the attentional and memory areas, imaging techniques have been used in the EF area (Merkley et al., 2008). Young patients (6–9 years) were compared to a control group with regard to regional differences in gray-matter thickness. Significant cortical thinning was evident in the group post-TBI, and this was found to be related to EF outcome, in particular to working memory skills.

Social functioning. The manner in which a child operates within a social environment, by relying on social skills and interacting with others, is fundamental to the development and formation of lasting relationships and to effective participation within the community (Beauchamp & Anderson, 2010; Blakemore, 2010). Disruptions to social skill development can result in psychological distress, social isolation, and reduced self-esteem, all of which have major implications for quality of life. The unique impact of disruption as a result of early brain insult is still poorly understood, but it is likely to have dramatic effects as these skills are developing and emerging during childhood and adolescence. Such disruption in early life may interfere with the child's capacity to acquire and develop social skills. Children with TBI are at particular risk of social problems for a number of reasons, including vulnerability of the social brain network to the impact of TBI, as well as the nature of sequelae from injury (physical, communication, cognitive, behavioral, academic), which will hinder social competence and social interactions.

Early research reported that children with TBI had lower levels of self-esteem and adaptive behavior, higher levels of loneliness and behavioral problems (Andrews, Rose, & Johnson, 1998), and more difficulties in peer relationships (Bohnert, Parker, & Warschausky, 1997) than controls. For example, Yeates and colleagues (2004) examined social functioning in 109 children with TBI aged 6–12 versus an orthopedic injury comparison group. They showed that parents of children with moderate to severe TBI reported their child to have poor social and behavioral functioning. In some cases, social skills deteriorated with time. These findings are consistent with previous studies utilizing smaller samples (Andrews, Rose, & Johnson, 1998). Although just beginning to emerge as a research focus, long-term outcome studies are beginning to identify links between poor social function following child TBI and persisting social maladjustment and reduced quality of life (Anderson, Catroppa, Morse, Haritou, & Rosenfeld, 2010; Cattelani, Lombardi, Brianti, & Mazzucchi, 1998).

Social adjustment. The majority of studies examining social skills following child TBI have focused on social adjustment and have used broad-band parent questionnaires, such as those tapping behavioral function—for example, the Child Behavior Checklist (Asarnow et al., 1991; Poggi, Liscio, Adduci, Galbiatti, et al., 2005)—or adaptive abilities—for example, the Vineland Adaptive Behavior Scales (e.g., Anderson, Catroppa, Morse, Haritou, & Rosenfeld, 2001; Fletcher, Ewing-Cobbs, Miner, Levin, & Eisenberg, 1990; Ganesalingham et al., 2011; Sparrow, Balla, & Cicchetti, 1984). Overall, these studies have been divided in their findings, with similar numbers reporting evidence that children and adolescents with TBI display greater social incompetence than control groups, as demonstrated by poorer parent ratings for socialization and communication skills (Fletcher et al., 1990; Max, Lindgren, Knutson, Pearson, et al., 1998; Levin, Hanten, & Li, 2009; Poggi et al., 2005), or, in contrast, no significant group differences (Anderson et al., 2001; Hanten et al., 2008; Papero, Prigatano, Snyder, & Johnson, 1993; Poggi et al., 2005). Some studies suggest that children with severe TBI are more impaired in socialization, communication, and/or social competence than children with milder injuries (Asarnow et al., 1991; Fletcher et al., 1990; Ganesalingam et al., 2011; Max et al., 1998; Yeates et al., 2004), but other studies failed to find these dose-response relationships (Papero et al., 1993).

Our research team recently conducted a study tracking 10-year functional outcomes from early TBI (age at injury < 7 years). Using parent report measures, we found differences between injury severity groups (mild, moderate, severe) for social skills and adaptive abilities, but with fewer severity effects for behavioral outcomes (Catroppa, Godfrey, Rosenfeld, Hearps, & Anderson, 2012). These findings highlight the persistence of social dysfunction in the long term post injury.

Social interaction. To study the interactional aspect of social function, Bohnert and colleagues (1997) and Prigatano and Gupta (2006) each investigated friendships of children who had sustained a TBI. Bohnert et al. (1997) employed both children and parents as respondents and found no differences between children with and without TBI in friendship networks or on the Friendship Quality Questionnaire (Parker & Asher, 1993). In contrast, Prigatano and Gupta (2006), using parent ratings, reported results that supported a dose-response relationship. Specifically, children with severe TBI reported fewer close friendships than children with moderate or mild TBI, and children with moderate TBI had fewer close friendships than children with mild TBI.

In an early study, Andrews and colleagues (1998) examined child and parent reports of social interactions and showed that children with TBI experienced higher levels of loneliness and a higher likelihood of aggressive or antisocial behaviors than controls. Similarly, Dooley, Anderson, Hemphill, and Ohan (2008) investigated aggressive responses in adolescents with a history of TBI, compared to a healthy control sample. These authors found that a history of TBI was related to higher rates of both reactive and proactive aggression.

A recent review (van Tol, Gorter, DeMatteo, & Meester-Delver, 2011) highlights the inconsistency of findings in the field of social interaction and participation after child TBI, with the authors arguing for research that incorporates mixed-methods approaches, in order to take advantage of both qualitative and quantitative information.

Social cognition. In contrast to social adjustment and social interaction, measurement within this domain is largely based on direct child assessments, although these are currently restricted to mostly experimental tools. This domain of social function has attracted a growing number of publications, which can be divided into the following areas: (a) social problem-solving, (b) social communication, and (c) social information processing (incorporating theory of mind and emotion perception).

a) Social problem-solving: Several recent studies have investigated social problem-solving in children and adolescents post-TBI. Hanten et al. (2008) and Janusz, Kirkwood, Yeates, and Taylor (2002) both used the Interpersonal Negotiation Strategies task (INS; Yeates, Schulz, & Selman, 1990), a child-based tool, to measure social problem-solving. The INS consists of several vignettes, which involve four social problem steps: defining the problem, generating alternative strategies, selecting and implementing a specific strategy, and evaluating outcomes. Using traditional and virtual reality versions of the INS, Hanten et al. (2008, 2011) found that children with a TBI scored significantly lower on social problem-solving from baseline through to one year post-TBI, with no differential improvement in performance one year after TBI in both the TBI and control groups. Similarly, Janusz et al. (2002) reported that children with TBI scored significantly lower on social problem-solving, being less able to generate solutions to social problems and less likely to choose optimal solutions.

Warschausky, Cohen, Parker, Levendosky, and Owen (1997) used a similar paradigm, the Social Problem-Solving Measure (Pettit, Dodge, & Brown, 1988), to assess solutions to social problems in children aged 7 and 13 years. Children with TBI provided significantly fewer peer-entry solutions in social engagement situations than control children, but the groups did not differ with regard to the number of solutions to peer provocations. In a study by our team (Muscara et al., 2008), we investigated the relationship between executive function and social function 10 years following child TBI, extending the work of Yeates et al. (2004), which had proposed that social problem-solving is a mediator between neurocognitive function and social skills, rather than a direct link. We identified greater executive dysfunction associated with less sophisticated social problem-solving skills and poorer social outcomes. Further, the maturity of social problem-solving skills was found to mediate the relationship between executive function and social outcomes in TBI. This study provided the first empirical evidence for a link between executive and social skills in the context of childhood acquired brain injury, due to the mediating link of social problem-solving.

b) Social communication: This domain of social function refers specifically to the child's ability to draw meaning from complex language. Tasks tapping these "pragmatic language" skills include aspects of cognitive function—for example, working memory and executive function, as well as abilities more commonly regarded as social cognition, such as the identification of irony and sarcasm in conversation and the ability to draw inferences from linguistic information and to distinguish truth from falsehoods (Turkstra, Dixon, & Baker, 2004; Turkstra, Williams, Tonks, & Frampton, 2008). Using the Video Social Inference Test with a group of adolescents with TBI, Turkstra et al. (2008) demonstrated that child TBI is associated with poorer identification of sarcasm and irony and greater difficulties interpreting inference in both photographs and stories. Dennis and colleagues have reported similar findings with younger children, showing deficits in understanding deceptive emotions, literal truth, irony, and deceptive praise (Dennis, Guger, Roncadin, Barnes, & Schachar, 2001; Dennis, Agostino, Taylor, Bigler, et al., 2013).

c) Social information processing: Studies investigating social information processing have focused primarily on theory of mind (ToM) and emotion perception in school-aged children and adolescents. For example, Turkstra et al. (2004, 2008) measured ToM in adolescents with TBI using a "second-order belief" task (i.e., requiring the ability to understand what one person thinks about another) and a pragmatic judgment test. They found that, in contrast to healthy controls, adolescents with TBI were deficient in judging whether a speaker was talking at the listener's level and in recognizing whether an individual was monopolizing a conversation. In contrast, the TBI group performed similarly to controls on a "first-order belief" task, such as identifying a good listener, as well as recognizing a faux pas and understanding pragmatic inferences in the Strange Stories test.

Walz and colleagues (2010) also examined ToM in a group of children who sustained TBI between 3 and 5 years of age and found few differences between children with TBI and controls. These authors raised the concern that, since ToM skills would be emerging in normally developing children at the time these children sustained their injuries, their results required follow-up. Of note, this group has recently studied a similar group of children who sustained their injuries slightly later (5–7 years) and demonstrated significant problems on ToM tasks, particularly for children with severe TBI. These studies highlight the need for a developmental perspective and the importance of taking into account both age at injury and age at assessment when interpreting study findings.

Children and adolescents with TBI have also been reported to have more difficulty recognizing emotions than controls. Tonks et al. (2009) found that children with a TBI were worse than control children at recognizing emotions expressed in the eyes, but they showed equivalent competence when recognizing facial emotions, suggesting that adding context assisted social information processing.

In summary, the weight of evidence indicates that children sustaining TBI are at elevated risk of experiencing social deficits, including social adjustment, social interaction, and social cognition. These problems persist long after insult. Further work is needed to describe the potential impact of injury-related factors (e.g., severity, age at insult) and environmental influences on these social consequences.

Functional Outcomes

Educational

The challenges of everyday functioning include the ability to progress in an educational setting. School placement has often been used as an indicator of educational performance following TBI, with re-entry often requiring modifications to assist children (Carney & Porter, 2009). As one would expect, reports have shown that children with moderate to severe TBI are more likely to present with greater difficulties in the years following the injury, with a weakness in school readiness skills, and therefore require special assistance (Stallings, Ewing-Cobbs, Francis, & Fletcher, 1996; Taylor et al., 2008). Kinsella and colleagues (1995, 1997) have reported that at one year post-injury, children with moderate to severe TBI were more likely to require special assistance at school, with 7 out of 10 children with severe injuries, and 2 out of 5 with moderate injuries, receiving special education two years post-injury. More recently, Hawley and colleagues (2004) showed that, regardless of injury severity, half their pediatric sample had a reading age one or more years below their chronological age, and one-third were two or more years below, therefore requiring special education in this area. In support of these findings, parents have also reported educational difficulties, although focusing on poorer health-related quality of life in the school domain (Erickson, Montague, & Gerstle, 2010).

Outcomes in the educational area have been researched within months to a year post-injury (Berger-Gross & Shackelford, 1985; Slater & Kohr, 1989). Findings have shown that children who had sustained a closed-head injury were functioning lower in areas including spelling, mathematics, reading, and word recognition in comparison to their peers, with poorer arithmetic skills linked to severity of injury. In a study conducted by Catroppa and Anderson (1999b), educational skills were investigated in a group of children injured between the ages of 8–12, at two years post-injury. Results showed that educational difficulties were present up to 24 months following moderate to severe traumatic brain injury. A dose-response relationship was found for listening comprehension and arithmetic, but not for reading accuracy and spelling, suggesting factors other than severity of injury influenced recovery of these skills over time. Raghubar, Barnes, Prasad, Johnson, and Ewing-Cobbs (2013) compared mathematical outcomes in children with moderate to severe injury to orthopedic controls at 2 and 24 months post-injury, with a focus on the role of working memory to math outcomes. It was found that children with TBI did not have deficits in math fact retrieval, but that verbal working memory mediated group differences on math calculations and applied problems.

A more in-depth investigation of reading skills following childhood head injury was undertaken by Barnes, Dennis, and Wilkinson (1999). Using a developmental perspective, it was hypothesized that following a TBI in childhood, younger children should be at the highest risk for difficulties in acquiring the basics of reading, such as word decoding. For those injured in middle childhood, the risk may be greatest for reading comprehension. Results showed that children who sustained injuries during preschool or early primary years were most at risk for difficulties in both decoding and comprehension skills. Children injured between 6.5 and 9 years performed better than younger children but more poorly than an older group of children.

With a focus on reading skills, Ewing-Cobbs et al. (2004, 2006) followed up children from time of injury until five to eight years post-injury, in a moderate to severe group injured between 4 and 71 months of age. Children with severe TBI showed persistent deficits in reading decoding, reading comprehension, spelling, and arithmetic. Furthermore, statistical analyses showed increases over time in achievement scores for children injured at an older age in comparison to those injured at a younger age. Reading accuracy, spelling, and arithmetic skills were also investigated at a mean follow-up interval of 6.8 years post-injury (Catroppa et al., 2005b) in children who had sustained a mild, moderate, or severe TBI, with an emphasis on age at injury: "young" age at injury (3–7 years) and "old" age at injury (8–12 years). Though a dose-response relationship for severity was evident for the young group on educational measures, this was not always the case for the older group, where it was suggested that pre-injury academic skills may play a role. Furthermore, reading ability was more compromised in the children injured at a younger age (Catroppa & Anderson, 1999b).

Behavioral/Adaptive Functions

Fletcher, Ewing-Cobbs, Miner, Levin, and Eisenberg (1990) found that children who sustained severe head injuries displayed a decline in adaptive functioning, whereas those with mild to moderate injuries did not deviate from average levels of functioning. More recently, a number of papers have emerged investigating diverse aspects of functional outcome following child TBI. Wells, Minnes, and Phillips (2009) investigated social/behavioral and functional outcomes and concluded that desired outcomes were dependent on developmental, severity, and family factors. Chapman and colleagues (2010) also reported poorer outcomes for those sustaining a severe injury with regard to externalizing problems, a result supported by Poggi et al. (2005) when comparing TBI and tumor survivors. Fay et al. (2009) investigated children who sustained a moderate or severe injury and compared them to an orthopedic control group with regard to long-term functional deficits. It was found that though functional deficits were evident up to four years post-injury, in two out of five children following severe injury, that outcome was also determined by variables including environmental factors and premorbid functioning. Yeates et al. (2010) also investigated outcomes such as behavioral adjustment, adaptive functioning and social competence, and the role of the family environment. The authors concluded that, though the family environment does moderate outcome, this influence may weaken over time for those children who sustained a severe injury.

Gerring and Wade (2012) reported that new-onset conduct disorder (CD) and disruptive symptoms are consequences of pediatric TBI at one year post-injury. Recently, Li and Liu (2012) published a systematic review with a focus on behavioral outcomes following pediatric TBI between 1990 and 2012. Findings revealed that up to 50% of children post brain-injury are at risk for behavior problems and disorders. Problems emerged shortly after the injury or several years later and persisted or worsened over time. These impairments were found to be modulated by the family environment, suggesting the need for intervention with a family focus (Wade, Cassedy, Walz, Taylor, et al., 2011).

Psychiatric

Investigating the severely injured children, Brown, Chadwick, Shaffer, Rutter, and Traub (1981) reported that there was also a marked increase in psychiatric disorders in this group of children following a brain injury. More recently, Massagli et al. (2004) showed that, at three years post-injury, even children with mild TBI were at significantly increased risk of psychiatric illness, particularly ADHD, with prior psychiatric problems a significant contributor. Even more recently, Gerring and Wade (2012) reported that the pre-injury prevalence of conduct disorder in the TBI sample was significantly higher than in a reference population and that the incidence of new-onset conduct disorder was also significantly higher than in a reference group. With regard to neuropsychiatric/emotional conditions post-injury, a review (Kim, Lauterbach, Reeve, Arciniegas, et al., 2007) indicated a gap in the literature in this area, but results suggested depression and post-traumatic amnesia are evident (Timonen, Miettunen, Hakko, Zitting, et al., 2002), with aggression, emotional difficulties, and conduct problems also present in this population (Dooley et al., 2008; Noggle & Pierson, et al., 2010; Tonks et al., 2009). Additionally, Max, Kaetley, Wilde, Bigler, et al. (2011) found that children who developed a novel anxiety disorder post-TBI were significantly younger than those who did not and that such problems were related to other new-onset difficulties of depression and personality change, with irritability seen as a key contributor.

Considering an adolescent age group post-TBI, Peterson et al. (2013) investigated internalizing behavior problems in adolescents across all severity levels, at one to six months post-injury. Parent ratings on the Child Behavior Checklist were within the average range, but adolescent ratings indicated an elevated risk of internalizing problems. Clinically significant internalizing symptoms were reported by a quarter of the adolescent sample. Parent psychopathology and female gender were predictive of adolescent outcome. In a paper concerned with the very long-term outcome of child TBI survivors, it was found that depression, anxiety, and poorer quality of life are clearly evident in this population in adulthood (Anderson et al., 2009).

Quality of Life (QoL)

As children mature post-TBI and develop into adolescents and young adults, quality of life (QoL) has emerged as an important functional domain to assess. QoL is often conceptualized as a multidimensional construct, and Dijkers (2004) provides a summary of its components. When the specific construct of health-related quality of life (HRQoL) was investigated, it was found that individuals with TBI scored lower than they did pre-injury and were poorer than comparison groups, differences were evident between participant and parent ratings, and post-concussive symptoms were linked to poorer QoL (Dijkers, 2004; Erickson et al., 2010; Gabbe et al., 2010, 2011; Green et al., 2012, 2013; Moran et al., 2012; Souza et al., 2007). In particular, Rivara et al. (2011) reported that, in children with moderate or severe TBI, as well as children with mTBI including an intracranial hemorrhage, a long-term reduction in QoL was evident, and this included participation in activities, quality of communication, and self-care.

A recent systematic review of children and adolescents post-TBI (Di Battista, Soo, Catroppa, & Anderson, 2012) aimed to further clarify the nature of HRQoL in survivors of pediatric TBI. Of 419 articles identified, 9 met inclusion criteria and were analyzed in the review. Four studies reported good QoL, and five reported poor QoL. The difference between good and poor QoL was statistically significant due to TBI severity, timing of outcome assessment, and definition of QoL. It was found that good outcomes were contingent on milder injuries, proxy reporting, and early assessment ($\leq$ 6 months), whereas poor outcomes were associated with more severe injuries and later assessment ($\geq$ 1 year). Swanson et al. (2012) extended these findings by reporting an association between CT results in children post-TBI and QoL at 12 months post-imaging. Taking a longer-term perspective, Anderson et al. (2009) found that poorer QoL in adult survivors of child TBI was also associated with low levels of perceived independence, younger age at injury, failure to complete high school, and psychological problems.

Trajectory of Outcomes Following Child TBI

As indicated by research concerned with outcomes following child TBI, children have been investigated at various time points and ages, and therefore the recovery/trajectory of skills over time post-injury is of much importance. Below are some examples from our laboratory (Figures 7.1–7.4). Figure 7.1 shows recovery in the area of attention in a group of children injured between the ages of 8 and 12 years, showing the role of severity of injury on outcome up to 24 months post-injury. Figures 7.2–7.4 illustrate the vulnerability of children injured between the ages of 1 and 7 years in areas including memory, adaptive, and behavioral domains, and educationally, with the severe group generally performing below the level of the control children and those with a lesser injury (Figures adapted from Anderson et al., 2004;

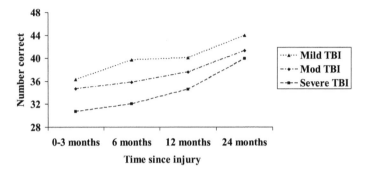

FIGURE 7.1

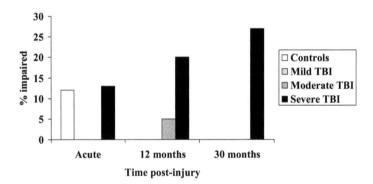

FIGURE 7.2

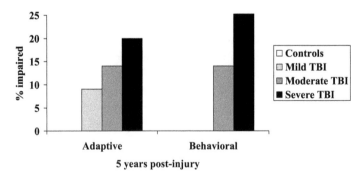

FIGURE 7.3

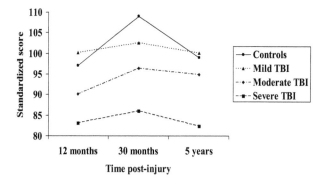

FIGURE 7.4

2005; Catroppa & Anderson, 2003; 2008; 2011). Longitudinal data support the vulnerability of skills that are emerging or developing at the time of injury. The data highlight the fact that some deficits may not be evident until a particular skill is expected to come online developmentally and that though children may improve and show developmental gains over time in some skill areas, they still remain below the level of same-aged peers or those with lesser injury (Beauchamp et al., 2011; Catroppa et al., 2007; Anderson et al., 2009).

Predictors of Outcome
(refer to Table 7.2 for summary of predictors)

Injury Factors

Indices including loss of consciousness (LOC), post-traumatic amnesia (PTA), neurological signs, and evidence of brain injury on imaging have been used to measure the severity of injury following child TBI. The Glasgow Coma Scale (GCS; Teasdale & Jennett, 1974), which is widely used as a measure of the depth and duration of impaired consciousness and assesses three aspects of behavior—eye opening, motor responses, and verbal responses—has been reported to be a predictor of outcome in both cognitive and functional domains, but also predictive of later parenchymal change (Ghosh et al., 2009). Post-traumatic amnesia (PTA) has also been argued to be a useful measure of the severity of diffuse brain damage (Rutter, Chadwick, & Shaffer, 1983), in which, following return to consciousness, there may follow a period of time during which recent events are not recalled reliably or accurately. The presence of neurological signs is an indicator of a moderate to severe TBI and may include hemiparesis, poor motor control, post-injury seizures, and hearing loss.

Imaging techniques (e.g., computed tomography, magnetic resonance imaging, diffusion weighted imaging, diffusion tensor imaging, susceptibility-weighted imaging, magnetic resonance spectroscopy) as presented in Chapter 5, and their methods of quantification (Bigler et al., 2010), are also important in detecting brain injury, from the identification of fractures to microscopic lesions and pathophysiological changes (Babikian et al., 2006, 2009; Beauchamp, Ditchfield, Babl, et al., 2011; Bigler & Maxwell, 2011; Chertkoff Walz, Cecil, Wade, & Michaud, 2008; Chu, Wilde, Hunter, McCauley, et al., 2010; Ewing-Cobbs et al., 2008; Galloway, Tong, Ashwal, Oyoyo, & Obenaus, 2008; Hunter et al., 2012; Kim & Gean, 2011; Le & Gean, 2009; Levin et al., 2008; Ljungqvist, Nilsson, Ljundberg, Sorbo, et al., 2011; Miles, Grossman, Johnson, Babb, et al., 2008; Provenzale, 2010; Suskauer & Huisman, 2009; Wilson, Wiedmann, Hadley, Condon, et al., 1988; Yuan et al., 2007). Though these indices of injury severity (as well as hypertension and high blood pressure) have been found to be successful predictors of impairment in physical, cognitive, social, educational, and functional domains following child TBI (Anderson et al., 2010; Beauchamp et al., 2009; Catroppa & Anderson, 1999b; Chertkoff Walz et al., 2008; Dennis et al., 1996; Fay et al., 2009; Fletcher, Ewing-Cobbs, Miner, Levin, & Eisenberg, 1990; Gale & Prigatano, 2010; Horneman & Emanuelson, 2009; Kinsella et al.,1997; Levin et al., 1987; Merkley et al., 2008; Salorio, Slomine, Guerguerian, Christensen, et al., 2008; Wilde et al., 2006), the search continues for further biomarkers (e.g., serum biomarkers such as calcium-binding protein S100B, neuron specific enolase NSE, myelin basic protein MBP) to diagnose and direct treatment following brain injury (Guerguerian, Milly Lo, & Hutchison, 2009; Pardes Berger, Beers, Rochichi, Wiesman, & Adelson, 2007; Sandler, Figaji, & Adelson; 2009; Shore, Berger, Varma, Janesco, et al., 2007; Stocchetti & Longhi, 2010).

Developmental Factors

From the literature on outcome following child TBI, it is clear that developmental aspects are implicated in the recovery and status of skills in the acute and longer-term stages post-TBI. Though it is outside the scope of this chapter to discuss the developmental trajectory of skills in the areas of attention (Betts, McKay, Maruff, & Anderson, 2006; Rebok et al., 1997), memory (Gomez-Perez & Ostrosky-Solis, 2006; Levin, Eisenberg, Wigg, & Kobayashi, 1982; Levin, High, Ewing-Cobbs, Fletcher, et al., 1988), EF (Anderson et al., 2001), and functional skills (Barnes, Dennis, & Wilkinson, 1999), it is important to note that these skills develop at different rates. From a developmental perspective, injury at an early age may affect cognitive skills developing at the time of injury, and skills yet to develop or reach maturity, with earlier-developing skills more consolidated and less vulnerable to childhood injury (Dennis, 1989; Dennis et al., 1995). Therefore, researchers have found injury age to be a reliable predictor of outcome (see Figure 7.5; adapted from Anderson et al., 2005b), with earlier injury often linked with poorer outcome on cognitive measures (Anderson & Moore, 1995; Anderson et al., 2005b; Donders & Warschausky, 2007; Johnson, DeMatt, & Salorio, 2009; Niedzwecki,

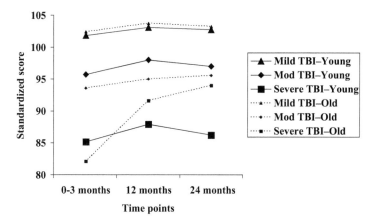

FIGURE 7.5

Marwitz, Ketchum, Cifu, et al., 2008; Prigatano & Gray, 2008). Age at injury has also been reported to be a significant predictor of emotional outcome following TBI (Senathi-Raja, Ponsford, & Schonberger, 2010). These researchers found that within a broad age range at time of injury (16–81 years), long-term emotional outcome was related to an interaction of age at injury and time post-injury, with poorer emotional outcome evident in younger individuals (16–27 years at injury) at longer time post-injury (14–22 years post-injury).

Environmental and Family Factors

McKinlay et al. (2010) reported that, prior to injury, certain factors predisposed a child to experience a TBI. It was found that being a male, number of adverse events in the family, and a punitive parenting style were all related to an increased likelihood of a TBI event occurring. Post-injury, socioeconomic status (SES), and family functioning/environment have been found to affect and predict cognitive, behavioral, and functional outcomes (Anderson et al., 2001; Bedell, 2008; Gerrard-Morris, Taylor, Yeates, Walz, et al., 2009; Rivara, Jaffe, Polissar, Fay, et al., 1994; Taylor, Drotar, Wade, Yeates, et al., 1995; Taylor et al., 2008; Wetherington, Hooper, Keenan, Nocera, et al., 2010; Yeates et al., 2004), suggesting a role for factors outside of the injury or developmental aspects of the child. Family cohesion (Rivara et al., 1994) and the quality of the home environment (Gerrard-Morris et al., 2009) have been found to underlie better outcome, while lower levels of SES have been linked with poorer outcome (Bijur, Goulding, Haslum, & Kurzon, 1988; Coster, Haley, & Baryza, 1994). In a recent paper, Yeates et al. (2010) investigated whether the family environment moderates psychosocial outcome in young children following TBI. It was found that though the family environment does moderate the outcome of young children, this influence was not consistent across time in those with severe injuries. Chapman et al. (2010) reported that predictors of significant behavior problems include low SES, family dysfunction, and permissive parenting, with Woods, Catroppa, Barnett, and Anderson (2011) further supporting the role of parental disciplinary patterns and behavior problems following child TBI.

Looking at parental characteristics, Wade, Chertkoff Walz, Carey, and Williams (2008) reported that parents of children with TBI exhibited fewer warm responses and made more directive statements during a given task in comparison to parents of uninjured children. These results suggested that child behavior post-TBI and parent responses (stress, depression, etc.) may have a reciprocal effect, causing dysfunction within the family system (Benn & McColl, 2004; Norup, Siert, & Lykke Mortensen, 2010; Stancin, Wade, Walz, Yeates, & Taylor, 2008), with families of children with severe injury experiencing long-standing burden, especially when supports were not available (Josie, Peterson, Burant, Drotar, et al., 2008; Wade, Wolfe, Maines Brown, & Pestian, 2005).

As becomes evident when reading the literature, it is often difficult to tease out a specific predictor for an indicated outcome or in fact across diverse outcomes. A combination of severe injury and social disadvantage have been found to be particularly detrimental to recovery following early brain insult (Breslau, 1990; Taylor et al., 1995). Wells et al. (2009) reported that age at injury and environmental factors were both significant predictors of social and functional outcomes but, in addition, that clinical expertise with regard to clinical rating of injury severity accounted for much of the variance in outcomes.

Premorbid Factors

Premorbid factors also play a part in the acute and longer-term outcome (Johnson, DeMatt, & Salorio, 2009; Kaldoja & Kolk, 2012) in cognitive and behavioral areas for children across injury severity. In a sample of children following mild TBI, Ponsford and colleagues (1999) found a clear relationship between pre-injury learning skills and post-injury behavioral difficulties. Psychiatric and emotional problems have also been reported to increase post-injury for children where such problems were present pre-injury (Brown, Chadwick, Shaffer, Rutter, & Traub, 1981; Gerring et al., 2009; Rutter, Chadwick, & Shaffer, 1983).

Genetic Factors

More recently, researchers have also been interested in the role of genetics in recovery from child TBI. Apolipoprotein E (ApoE) is a protein that plays a role in the recovery of injured nerve tissue (Wright, Hu, Silverman, Tsaih, et al., 2003). In a paper investigating this protein in a normative sample of mother–child dyads, it was suggested that those carrying the E4 allele (other common alleles are known as E2 and E3) had an advantage with regard to early brain development. Other researchers have therefore been interested in the relationship of this gene to recovery from brain injury. It has been reported that E4 appears to be deleterious post-injury

TABLE 7.2 Predictors of Outcome from Childhood Brain Injury

Factors found to contribute to outcome from childhood brain injury

Injury factors
  Severity (mild, moderate, severe)
  Nature (diffuse, focal)
  Disability (post-traumatic epilepsy, neurological signs, physical/speech impairment)
Developmental factors
  Age at injury
  Developmental stage
Pre-injury factors
  Pre-injury child function: cognitive ability, personality
  Pre-injury family factors: family function, parents' mental health
  Gender
Environmental factors
  Socioeconomic status
  Access to resources—educational, rehabilitation
Genetic factors
  Apolipoprotein gene (ApoE)

Source: Adapted from Anderson & Catroppa (2006).

in adults, but that it could be protective, with regard to brain development, in young children (Blackman, Worley, & Strittmatter, 2005). However, such results are inconclusive, with some findings suggesting the E4 allele increases the risk of poor clinical outcome (Dardiotis, Fountas, Dardioti, Xiromerisiou, et al., 2010). Looking specifically at mild TBI in children between the ages of 8 and 15, Moran et al. (2009) compared children with and without the E4 allele. It was found that those with the E4 allele performed better on a test of constructional skill, but no further differences were found on other neuropsychological tests, nor on measures of post-concussive symptoms. It was concluded that the E4 allele was not a consistent predictor of outcomes following childhood mild TBI.

As summarized by Gerring and Wade (2012), the number, type, and interaction of risk factors, protective factors, and recovery all play a role in predicting outcome following child TBI.

Conclusions

It is clear that a TBI in childhood may have a number of cognitive, behavioral, adaptive, and social consequences. Often, poorer outcomes are evident in those with more severe injury; however, this may not always be the case, as seen in behavioral outcomes. Furthermore, difficulties in the acute period often persist in the longer term. Prediction of outcome, in order to identify those children at risk in the longer term, is often difficult, though pre-injury status, injury severity, age at injury, and family characteristics often play a role.

8

THE EVOLUTION OF CHILD TBI INTO ADULTHOOD

Introduction

The management, assessment, follow-up, and rehabilitation of child TBI is beginning to be well-established, as outlined in previous sections of this text. At the other
end of the age spectrum there also currently exists a substantial body of evidence
describing the consequences of adult TBI, with findings indicating significant
problems (physical, cognitive, educational, vocational, psychological) persisting
even several decades post-injury and including social and psychiatric disturbance
(Engberg & Teasdale, 2004; Hoofien, Gilboa, Vakil, & Donovick, 2001). In contrast,
the impact of child TBI in the very long term, as children and adolescents develop
into adults, is poorly understood. From a clinical perspective, the absence of clear
and reliable predictors of outcome make providing families with an accurate picture of their child's health status and abilities in future years speculative at best.
Some clinicians and researchers argue for the presence of serious and persisting
sequelae, even after mild TBI, while others argue that the increased plasticity of the
young brain will override any potential sequelae observed in the short to medium
term post-injury. In recent years, the debate opposing proponents of plasticity
theory (the idea that the young brain is flexible and able to reorganize and that
TBI at young ages results in few deficits; Kennard, 1936) to those who believe
early brain injuries result in worse outcomes (Anderson et al., 2005b; Anderson,
Spencer-Smith, et al., 2009; Beauchamp, Dooley, & Anderson, 2010) because of the
increased vulnerability of the developing brain has fueled contemporary notions
of the very long term consequences of child TBI. Unfortunately, opportunities to
follow children with TBI into adulthood are limited both clinically and scientifi-
cally. Perceptions that children will recover well from TBI, and limited availability
of financial and health resources, mean that usually only the most severely injured
patients will receive medical services in the long term. From a research perspective,

only a handful of studies have followed survivors of child TBI into adulthood, with somewhat conflicting results, possibly due to inherent methodological problems of longitudinal research, including sample attrition and bias and changes in diagnostic and treatment approaches over time. However, the limited evidence available from long-term studies of child TBI does support the notion that treatment and management of the head-injured child and family requires long-term involvement. Health professionals have a role to play in maintaining an understanding of the patient's ongoing difficulties and evolving skills. They also inform families and the wider community of the cognitive and behavioral implications of TBI; liaise with teachers, rehabilitation workers, and employers to design academic and vocational interventions and behavior management programs; and provide counseling with respect to adjustment issues for the brain-injured patient, family, and significant others.

Adult Outcome of Child TBI

Though only a few studies have reported on adult outcome after mild TBI in childhood, results are consistent and suggest very few major long-term neurobehavioral consequences (Hessen, Nestvold, & Anderson, 2007; McKinlay, Dalrymple-Alford, Horwood, & Fergusson, 2002), although psychological problems appear to be more common (Hessen, Anderson, & Nestvold, 2008). In contrast, there is a growing body of research addressing adult outcome from more severe TBI in childhood. Even in these studies, reports of gross neurobehavioral impairment are relatively rare, and most survivors tend to manage adequately through their school years (Jonsson, Horneman, & Emanuelson, 2004; Nybo, Sainio, & Muller, 2004), although some may show specific long-term medical and physical problems (Klonoff, Clark, & Klonoff, 1993; Koskiniemi, Kyykka, Nybo, & Jarho, 1995), as well as cognitive deficits and vocational and educational difficulties, as described below (e.g., Hoofien et al., 2001; Jonsson et al., 2004; Klonoff et al., 1993; Nybo & Koskiniemi, 1999).

Cognitive Outcome

Though cognitive deficits usually improve during the two first years post-injury in children, recovery plateaus after this time, and remaining deficits may continue to affect functioning into adulthood (van Heugten et al., 2006; Yeates, Taylor, Wade, Drotar, et al., 2002). Where cognitive problems are detected in the very long term after child TBI, they tend to be subtle and to affect more dynamic cognitive domains, such as attention, memory and executive function, and processing speed (Asikainen, Nybo, Muller, Sarna, & Kaste, 1999; Beauchamp et al., 2011; Cattelani, Lombardi, Brianti, & Mazzucchi, 1998; Nybo & Koskiniemi, 1999). As a more global indicator of cognitive ability, intellectual function appears to improve to low-average-to-average levels in the very long term (10 years) even after severe child TBI, suggesting that children with TBI do make developmental gains in the long term (Anderson,

Godfrey, Rosenfeld, & Catroppa, 2011). These findings are supported by a retrospective study of adult survivors of child TBI, which similarly found good (average) intellectual outcomes (Anderson, Brown, Newitt, & Hoile, 2011).

Educational and Vocational Outcome

Research findings demonstrate that injuries sustained during childhood affect vocational outcome. Ewing-Cobbs and colleagues (2006) found that almost 50% of patients with TBI failed a school grade or required placement in special education classrooms, and the odds of unfavorable academic performance were 18 times higher for patients versus controls. Such poor academic success has significant implications for later vocational outcomes. Koskiniemi, Kyykka, Nybo, and Jarho (1995) further showed that following preschool TBI, normal school performance or intelligence does not necessarily translate to good vocational outcome, suggesting that almost any child with brain injury may be at risk for professional problems or unemployment. In contrast to the finding that intellectual functions were spared in adult survivors of child TBI, Anderson and colleagues found that those with severe TBI were more likely to have educational and employment problems (Anderson, Brown, et al., 2011). Academic difficulties appear to persist in the long term after child TBI regardless of age of injury, especially in those with moderate and severe injuries (Catroppa et al., 2009a). The same study found that significant predictors of word reading and spelling abilities in the long term include acute Full Scale Intellectual Quotient (FSIQ), suggesting that though intellectual function may recover in the very long term, earlier difficulties in this broad domain affect educational achievement. Acute IQ and injury severity both predict arithmetic outcomes in the long term.

Emotional, Social, and Behavioral Outcome

There is increasing evidence that after child TBI, social and emotional deficits increase and persist into adulthood, having unfavorable effects on daily living, ability to engage in work and social activities, and coping with adult responsibilities. These difficulties may be exacerbated by accumulated failures and frustrations throughout development, which may cause survivors to withdraw from regular work and leisure activities and exacerbate significant emotional problems. Available research has identified social and psychological/psychiatric problems as being highly represented complaints among adult survivors of child TBI and can include social maladjustment and isolation, poor quality of life, depression, attention deficits, and family problems, with an association between pre-injury factors and injury severity and presence of difficulties (Anderson, Brown, Newitt, & Hoile, 2009; Cattelani et al., 1998; Hoofien et al., 2001; Klonoff et al., 1993).

TBI is also associated with a high rate of emotional and behavioral problems in adulthood, including increased anxiety, depression, and poor coping skills (Anson &

Ponsford, 2006; Draper, Ponsford, & Schonberger, 2007; Ponsford, Draper, & Schonberger, 2008). Although some patients suffer from lifetime psychiatric disorders, there is also evidence for the emergence of novel disorders, particularly following severe injury during childhood. Bloom and colleagues (2001) reported that attention-deficit/hyperactivity disorder and depression are the most common novel diagnoses, though a variety of psychiatric diagnoses may be present, with 74% of disorders persisting in 48% of injured children. Post-injury personality disorders have also been identified in a high proportion of TBI survivors (66%), though there does not appear to be a TBI-specific personality syndrome, given that common post-TBI disorders range across borderline, avoidant, paranoid, obsessive-compulsive, and narcissistic personality types (Hibbard, Bogdany, Uysal, Kepler, et al., 2000).

In our own prospective longitudinal study, we found that adolescents and young adults who sustained TBI during early childhood demonstrated elevated risk of developing psychological problems following their transition into adulthood, with greatest problems for internalizing symptoms, such as depression, anxiety, and withdrawal (Rosema, Muscara, Anderson, Godfrey, Eren, & Catroppa, 2014).

Evidence is emerging that suggests a cognitive basis for some social problems after TBI, with studies reporting deficits in socio-cognitive skills, such as problem solving, theory of mind, empathy, and moral reasoning (e.g., Beauchamp, Dooley, & Anderson, 2013; Muscara, Catroppa, & Anderson, 2008b; Turkstra, Dixon, & Baker, 2004; Walz et al., 2010; Wood & Williams, 2008); however, the impact of these difficulties in adulthood is unknown. The adverse consequences of early brain injury in later life may be illustrated by the high prevalence of child TBI survivors (of all severity levels) in incarcerated juvenile centers (35%) (Kenny & Jennings, 2007) and in adult prisoners (up to 87%) (Leon-Carrion & Ramos, 2003; Slaughter, Fann, & Ehde, 2003; Timonen et al., 2002), indicating that TBI survivors could be at risk for exhibiting maladaptive behaviors, with serious legal implications later in life, though it is unclear what factors explain or are associated with such serious, maladaptive consequences.

At a global level, there is evidence that overall quality of life is affected in the very long term after severe TBI, with lower IQ and personality factors predicting outcome in this broad domain and suggesting a cumulative effect of cognitive and psychosocial factors on the capacity for child TBI survivors to benefit positively from work and leisure activities (Anderson, Brown, et al., 2011). Poor quality of life is associated with severe TBI, alongside low levels of perceived independence, younger age at injury, failure to complete high school (see educational and vocational outcomes), and psychological problems (Anderson, Brown, & Newitt, 2010).

Factors Influencing Adult Outcomes

Outcome from child TBI is highly variable, and a number of factors have been established as contributing to recovery, at least up to five years post-insult: injury severity and injury age, premorbid characteristics of the child, and psychosocial factors (Anderson et al., 2005b; Hessen et al., 2007; Koskiniemi et al., 1995). Other factors of potential importance include access to rehabilitation and other resources, child and family adjustment, and degree of residual disability (Anderson et al., 2005b; Yeates et al., 1997). The limited body of research addressing long-term effects of child TBI suggests that similar factors may be relevant for long-term outcome (Anderson et al., 2010; Anderson, Godfrey, et al., 2011; Hoofien, Vakil, Gilboa, Donovick, & Barak, 2002; Nybo & Koskiniemi, 1999), although the research emphasis to date has been almost entirely on injury-based predictors. Acute medical factors, such as the need for neurosurgical intervention and raised intracranial pressure, may also affect long-term outcomes (Aaro Jonsson, Smedler, Leis Ljungmark, & Emanuelson, 2009; Jagannathan, Okonkwo, Yeoh, Dumont, et al., 2008).

Assessment of Adult Outcomes

Neuropsychological assessment plays an important part in the diagnostic, recovery, and rehabilitation processes post-TBI, and the characteristics of such childhood assessments at the acute stage are described in Chapter 4. In the very long term, assessment tends to be more frequent for severely injured individuals who suffer serious deficits that significantly affect their ability to function in daily life. Ongoing assessment throughout adolescence and into adulthood may be necessary to track the development of cognition post-injury and to identify changing needs as the brain recovers and environmental demands change (e.g., reintegration to school or work). Survivors of child TBI may even appear to make a full recovery in the initial stages post-injury, with latent TBI symptoms emerging only months or even years after injury, as developmental milestones are attained (Giza & Prins, 2006). Neuropsychological assessment is of benefit throughout the life span. By the time individuals injured during childhood reach early adulthood, they are generally well aware of the lasting effects of their injury on various spheres of their lives. As they transition to adulthood, it may be necessary to re-evaluate their capacity to cope, both cognitively and emotionally, with new demands and responsibilities. For example, a change in employment may precipitate new challenges by tapping previously unused skills or by increasing cognitive demands. Difficulties in dealing with such changes may require an assessment to identify areas of dysfunction and how these may be compensated for, so that the individual can better manage his or her new environment.

Although some restoration of function may occur, the late appearance of cognitive and behavioral problems may be associated with a failure of particular brain regions (and their associated cognitive skills) to develop, either as a direct result of TBI or due to progressive atrophy or loss of neural activity (Giza, Mink, & Madikians, 2007; Giza & Prins, 2006). These processes may lead to atypical patterns of cognitive function due to structural and functional re-assignment in the injured brain, and therefore, neuropsychological outcomes after child TBI are also partially a function of brain plasticity. Accordingly, individuals who demonstrate similar performance levels on a particular test may in fact be relying on different neural substrates. This suggests that assessments in the long term should rely on refined methods capable of detecting subtle cognitive variations and compensation strategies. Long-term evaluation therefore requires an understanding of neural reorganization, maturation, and degeneration, as well as their interaction with developmental growth and experience (Anderson et al., 2005b).

The unique characteristics of adult outcomes of child TBI have consequences for the goal and structure of remote neuropsychological assessment, which must be considered as distinct from the early, post-acute, and developmental evaluations following injury and different from the acute assessment of mature adults who sustain injuries. Some of the objectives of these later assessments may include a) developing an up-to-date cognitive profile in keeping with the patient's environment; b) identifying chronic neuropsychological impairments; c) re-assessing cognitive, behavioral, and social functions in light of adult milestones and evolving roles and responsibilities; d) tailoring assessment to pinpoint subtle areas of dysfunction; e) generating cognitive strategies to assist with daily life; and f) investigating the potential effects of brain plasticity and the role of neural reorganization/recruitment for cognitive and behavioral function.

In keeping with a shift in goals, there is also a shift in focus when conducting neuropsychological assessments in adults with childhood injuries. As in the acute phase, testing in the long term remains an individualized undertaking, tailored to the needs and characteristics of the client; however, these types of evaluations have their own qualities. First, long-term follow-up assessments need to be specific and sensitive, as the major areas of difficulty for the patient will have been previously identified. Second, the clinician needs to be aware that subjective complaints and self-reports of daily functioning may be greatly influenced by compensatory strategies established over the years post-injury, as well as habituation to existing deficits. In this sense, a lack of subjective complaints may not accurately reflect absence of cognitive dysfunction (nor lack of insight), as adults may have developed adaptations and compensatory mechanisms that mask the nature and extent of existing problems. Third, age at injury is an important consideration, as it will affect the extent and nature of the neurocognitive skills likely to have been impacted by brain injury. Donders and Warschausky (2007) demonstrated that early-onset child TBI results in worse outcomes in higher-level cognitive skills and social integration than later "transition age" (17–21 years) injuries. The relative impact of TBI on cognitive and social skills is a function of the stage of development at injury; skills that are not yet solidified may be particularly vulnerable to trauma. Fourth, ongoing review of the impact of childhood TBI into adulthood may need to rely increasingly on measures that reflect real-life skills and behavior in order to address the daily impact of chronic TBI sequelae. There is increasing interest in the ecological validity of the neuropsychological assessment, though adequate measures are still scarce (Chaytor, Temkin, Machamer, & Dikmen, 2007;

Silver, 2000). Results obtained within the confines of a standard assessment need to be interpreted with a consideration of real-world environments, which can be chaotic and noisy, and hence more difficult for individuals with brain injuries to negotiate. Obtaining an adequate history and information from third parties can help paint an accurate picture of an individual's functioning in the real world (Sbordone, 2001).

Cognitive Assessment

The evaluation of cognitive function remains the cornerstone of neuropsychological assessment at any stage post-injury and at any age. Identifying mental strengths and weaknesses is of fundamental importance to providing individuals with brain injury and their families with an accurate depiction of their current abilities. Neuropsychological assessment in the long term following child TBI should continue to be based on individualized systemic evaluation of cognitive skills. Measurement of IQ is still useful to obtain an up-to-date representation of global intellectual functioning. In order to minimize overuse of full IQ scales, abbreviated IQ tools can be helpful (e.g., Wechsler Abbreviated Scale of Intelligence; Wechsler, 1999). Using standardized measures of cognitive function, particularly those that are applicable to wide age brackets, procures the advantage of providing scores that can be compared across the life span from one assessment to another, enabling the neuropsychologist to track change over time. However, practice effects should be considered when interpreting results from individuals exposed to multiple assessments over the years, particularly when these are conducted in a relatively short time span, even when efforts are made to use alternate forms of tests.

Specific cognitive domains of interest include attention, memory and learning, processing speed, executive function, visuospatial and visuomotor skills, language, reading, and mathematics. Though standardized assessments exist for most of these areas, the need for a more specific and subtle evaluation in the long term suggests that it will be beneficial for the clinician to carefully choose tests that are valid and reliable and that span child and adult age bands (see Lezak, Howieson, & Loring, 2004; Strauss, Sherman, & Spreen, 2006, for test reviews).

Vocational Assessment

Survivors of TBI in full-time employment demonstrate better intellectual capacities and fewer executive deficits (Lachapelle, Bolduc-Teasdale, Ptito, & McKerral, 2008; Nybo et al., 2004), as well as largely intact perceptual, complex visual processing, attention, and memory capacities (Lachapelle et al., 2008; Ownsworth & McKenna, 2004), suggesting that assessment of these skills is an important aspect of the neuropsychological evaluation of vocational outcomes. Though such cognitive factors are of fundamental importance in determining an individual's ability to undertake and maintain full-time work, research also shows that they cannot alone predict vocational outcome. Environmental demands, along with social and emotional factors, are also critical when determining the need for vocational rehabilitation and support (Guerin, Kennepohl, Leveille, Dominique, & McKerral, 2006; Johnstone, Hexum, & Ashkanazi, 1995; Mateer & Sira, 2006). Self-awareness, in particular, has been identified as an important factor in successful return to work and should therefore be considered to be related to vocational success (Shames, Treger, Ring, & Giaquinto, 2007).

Emotional, Social, and Behavioral Assessment

Yeates and colleagues (2004) suggest that behavioral, emotional, and social difficulties are related to executive abilities, pragmatic language, and social problem-solving skills, and these are important in determining social functioning throughout the life span post-TBI. Measures of social functioning are often limited to general, parent-based reports, which are not useful with adults. Few of the existing measures are standardized, and no appropriate tools exist for evaluating the long-term social implications of TBI into adulthood. Some measures that may be of use for evaluating adaptive, functional, and psychosocial outcomes in adults are the Community Integration Questionnaire (Willer, Ottenbacher, & Coad, 1994) and the Sydney Psychosocial Reintegration Scale (Tate, Hodgkinson, Veerabangsa, & Maggiotto, 1999). In addition, the Dysexecutive Questionnaire, part of the Behavioral Assessment of the Dysexecutive Syndrome (Wilson, Alderman, Burgess, Emslie, & Evans, 1996), can be useful for identifying everyday signs of executive problems, which may affect social and behavioral function.

Given the prevalence of both Axis I and Axis II psychiatric diagnoses following child TBI, an initial screening of such disorders, and of more general emotional and behavioral problems (e.g., Minnesota Multiple Personality Inventory–2; Hathaway & McKinley, 1989), can be useful when frank psychiatric problems are suspected. The need for further referral for full psychiatric evaluation can also be considered, using structured clinical interview techniques to complement the neuropsychological profile of cognitive, social, and emotional abilities.

Conclusions

Assessment of outcome in a variety of domains is important for the lifelong management of child-TBI-related dysfunction and for ongoing monitoring of recovery, adaptation, and compensation as a function of fluctuating environmental demands and responsibilities. Assessment of child TBI in adulthood is distinct from evaluation performed acutely, and it entails a number of challenges and particular considerations. Evaluation must make allowances for ongoing development and aging, reorganization of structure and function, compensatory mechanisms and habituation, practice effects, real-world functioning, changing life situations, and the demands of the current environment. Thorough assessment remains important, though there may be a shift in focus from cognitive domains to the evaluation of social, emotional, and behavioral problems, as well as vocational outcomes and adaptive capabilities. Continued collaboration with other health professionals, as well as ongoing referral to rehabilitation and intervention programs when needed, remains essential.

9

ACUTE MANAGEMENT OF CHILD TBI

Effective acute management of TBI is critical for minimizing secondary consequences of TBI, such as raised intracranial pressure, edema, and vascular disruption. Despite its importance, advances in care have been slow to emerge, and emergency care staff are limited by a surprising lack of evidence-based information regarding gold standard interventions. Though it is now well recognized that the developing brain is highly vulnerable to injury, much of the routine acute care management for child TBI is based largely on adult models.

The aims of this chapter are to (a) summarize the phases of acute management and rehabilitation for child TBI; (b) provide an overview of existing guidelines for the acute management of child TBI; (c) summarize current best practice in acute management of child TBI; and (d) comment on future directions in research on acute management.

Phases and Models for Management and Rehabilitation

The aim of acute medical management and rehabilitation is to obtain the best outcomes for children and adolescents following TBI. The goal is to reduce mortality and morbidity, by ensuring survival with as little residual neurological insult as possible. The two main goals of rehabilitation are to (a) reduce the everyday consequences of residual cognitive and behavioral impairments (i.e., disabilities) and (b) reduce the level of handicap (i.e., the extent to which these impairments impede successful re-entry into society), in part by promoting community reintegration (Chevignard, Brooks, & Truelle, 2010; Wilson, 2000). Rehabilitation of child TBI thus involves working with the family to understand as well as treat impairments and to identify the link between impairments and functional or everyday difficulties (Anderson & Catroppa, 2006; Ylvisaker et al., 2005). Rehabilitation has been described as involving three phases, from the acute stage to longer-term (Mazaux & Richer, 1998): (i) to provide sensory stimulation during coma and low-arousal states; (ii) to facilitate recovery of functioning and compensate for residual difficulties; and (iii) to facilitate successful re-entry into the community.

For rehabilitation to be successful, a multidisciplinary team is essential, in both acute and later stages of recovery, as is family involvement in the process (Anderson & Catroppa, 2006). Models of intervention are often based on theories of restitution or substitution. "Restitution" involves the restoration of function via re-establishment of impaired functions, presumably by restoration of damaged tissue. Potential mechanisms for restitution may include regeneration, sprouting, and denervation supersensitivity, and are often the focus during the acute stage of rehabilitation (Kolb & Gibb, 1999; Kolb & Wishaw, 1996; Rothi & Horner, 1983). "Substitution" focuses on functional adaptation and is more common in the longer-term post-injury, where intact abilities are utilized to "re-route" skills that have been disrupted. Two potential mechanisms for substitution are anatomical reorganization and behavioral compensation (Cicerone & Tupper, 1990; Kolb & Wishaw, 1996; Rothi & Horner, 1983; Sohlberg & Mateer, 1989). Developmental theory is also crucial to inform the timing of intervention during both acute and longer-term recovery, taking into account both medical considerations (i.e., optimal time for particular medications in the acute phase) and transitional considerations (i.e., difficulties most common in adolescence rather than early childhood post-TBI) (Anderson & Catroppa, 2006).

Guidelines for Acute Medical Management of TBI

A variety of guidelines have been published relevant to the acute management of child TBI (Adelson, Bratton, Carney, Chesnut, et al., 2003; Gabriel et al., 2002; Kochanek, Carney, & Adelson, 2012; National Institute for Health and Clinical Excellence, 2007). Most of the guidelines have been based largely on expert consensus, due to the lack of a strong empirical evidence base, and they often represent a simple downward extension of adult guidelines.

In the United States, the first edition of the *Guidelines for Medical Management of Severe Traumatic Brain Injury for Infants, Children, and Adolescents* was published in 2003 (Adelson et al., 2003). The guidelines contained no standards and included only eight guidelines, with four of those being proscriptive (e.g., corticosteroids should be avoided). The second edition of the guidelines, published in 2012, was more strongly focused on empirical evidence and less reliant on expert opinion than the first edition (Kochanek et al., 2012). The second edition does not contain any recommendations based on Class 1 evidence (i.e., high-quality randomized clinical trials), and it contains only four based on Class II (lower-quality RCTs and higher-quality clinical studies), with just one of those being supportive of a particular therapeutic approach. All remaining guidelines are based on Class III evidence (i.e., lower-quality observational studies).

Despite the weak evidence base, the development of guidelines for acute management likely is in part responsible for declines in mortality and morbidity associated with pediatric TBI (Haque & Enam, 2009). The guidelines reflect a focus on two primary goals in the management of pediatric TBI, which are (1) stabilization and prevention of secondary insult and (2) management of intracranial hypertension (Kochanek, 2005). Based on existing guidelines, pre-hospital and acute medical management currently seeks to avoid hypotension, hypoxemia, hyperthermia, and iatrogenic hyperventilation and to maintain optimal blood pressure, cerebral perfusion pressure (CPP), brain oxygenation, and intracranial pressure (ICP). What follows is a summary of best practice to achieve these goals, as reflected in current guidelines.

Pre-hospital Management

Effective pre-hospital management is critical to reducing the mortality and morbidity associated with moderate to severe child TBI. No comprehensive, pediatric-specific guidelines for pre-hospital management have been published, although both the National Institute for Health and Clinical Excellence (2007) guidelines from the United Kingdom and the first edition of the US guidelines (Adelson et al., 2003) touch on pre-hospital management. A comprehensive set of guidelines for pre-hospital management was published in the United States by the Brain Trauma Foundation (Gabriel et al., 2002), although they are not specific to children. The implementation of these guidelines has led to reductions in mortality and better outcomes (Watts, Hanfling, Waller, Gilmore, et al., 2004).

The goals of pre-hospital management are to stabilize patients for transportation, triage those with mass lesions and impending cerebral herniation, and prevent secondary brain insults (Stiver & Manley, 2008). First responders initially focus on the "ABCs" of trauma care (i.e., airway, breathing, circulation). Key components of care include establishing airway control to reduce hypoxemia, providing fluid resuscitation to manage shock and maintain blood pressure, and preventing fever (i.e., hyperthermia). Cervical immobilization is critical whenever spinal-cord injury is a possibility. Management of pain and agitation is also important, because they can result in increases in ICP (Hsiang, Chesnut, Crisp, Klauber, et al., 1994); sedation, analgesia, and neuromuscular blockade may be necessary in this context. With regard to airway control, research has addressed the choice of intubation versus non-invasive methods (e.g., bag mask). Although the Brain Trauma Foundation guidelines call for intubation (Gabriel et al., 2002), the first edition of the US guidelines for management of pediatric TBI did not find compelling evidence to favor one method over the other (Adelson et al., 2003).

The triage of mass lesions and impending cerebral herniation demands close attention to signs of potential herniation, including pupillary changes, hypertension, bradycardia, motor posturing, and declines in level of consciousness. If such signs are present, hyperventilation and administration of hypertonic saline or mannitol may be necessary prior to emergency neurosurgical intervention. Routine hyperventilation is avoided, however, because it can decrease cerebral blood flow.

Another critical decision in pre-hospital management is where to transport children with TBI for acute medical care. The first edition of the US guidelines (Adelson et al., 2003) called for the direct transportation of children with severe TBI to dedicated pediatric trauma centers. This recommendation was based on the results of several studies showing that children who are directly transferred to Level 1 Pediatric Trauma Centers have decreased mortality compared to children who are only transferred indirectly (Hulka, Mullins, Mann, Hedges, et al., 1997; Johnson & Krishnamurthy, 1996).

Acute Hospital Management

The acute hospital care of child TBI has largely the same goals as pre-hospital management, including reduction of secondary injury and management of intracranial hypertension (Bell & Kochanek, 2013; Kochanek, 2005). The original US guidelines (Adelson et al., 2003) contained a specific algorithm for the management of ICP that recommended first- and second-tier therapies. First-tier therapies included sedation and analgesia, CSF drainage, neuromuscular blockade, hyperosmolar therapy or mannitol, and mild hyperventilation. Second-tier therapies, to be considered if first-tier therapies fail, included lumbar craniospinal fluid (CSF) drainage, high-dose barbiturates, decompressive craniectomy (the removal of sections of the skull to treat intracranial hypertension or herniation), aggressive hyperventilation, and hypothermia. The second edition of the US guidelines does not contain a specific algorithm but retains a focus on ICP management, with guidelines addressing the following topics:

1. indications for ICP monitoring, which is recommended for children with severe TBI;
2. thresholds for treatment of intracranial hypertension;
3. thresholds for cerebral perfusion pressure;
4. hyperosmolar therapy, supporting the use of hypertonic saline to reduce ICP;
5. hypothermia, which should be avoided if delivered for only 24 hours or with rapid rewarming but can be considered in the presence of intracranial hypertension if provided for a longer period with gradual rewarming;
6. CSF drainage, which can be considered for managing increased ICP;
7. use of high-dose barbiturates, which can be considered in cases of intracranial hypertension;
8. decompressive craniectomy, which may be considered in children showing neurological deterioration, herniation, or refractory intracranial hypertension;
9. hyperventilation, which should not be used prophylactically but reserved for refractory intracranial hypertension;

10. corticosteroids, which are not recommended; and
11. analgesics, sedatives, and neuromuscular blockade, the uses of which are left largely to physician discretion, with recommendations for two specific agents.

Additional guidelines address advanced neuromonitoring (i.e., recommended threshold for partial pressure of brain-tissue oxygen—PbO_2—if it is monitored); neuroimaging (i.e., avoid routine repeat CT scan in the absence of neurological deterioration or increased ICP); nutrition (i.e., lack of support for an immune-modulating diet); and seizure prophylaxis (i.e., support for the consideration of phenytoin in treatment of early post-traumatic seizures).

As noted earlier, only four of the new US guidelines were based on Class II evidence, and only one of those, regarding hyperosmolar therapies, supported a specific therapeutic approach. The remaining Class II recommendations were all negative: avoid hypothermia to improve outcomes; proscribe corticosteroids; and negative evidence for immune-modulating diets. All other recommendations were based on Class III evidence, and even then the available evidence did not support definitive recommendations for multiple issues, including glycemic control, CSF drainage, and analgesics/sedatives/neuromuscular blockade. Clearly, substantially more research is needed to provide a strong evidence base for the acute management of pediatric TBI.

Despite specific recommendations in the US guidelines, considerable controversy continues regarding the role of both hypothermia and craniectomy. Hypothermia purportedly can reduce the impact of secondary brain insult associated with increased ICP and reduced CPP, thus improving long-term outcome (Alzaga, Cerdan, & Varon, 2007; Sahuquillo & Vilalta, 2007). Jiang and Yang (2007) reviewed more than 30 studies regarding the status of protective effects of mild to moderate hypothermia on children and adults post-TBI. They reported only one clinical trial of mild to moderate hypothermia that demonstrated no effect in patients with severe TBI, and they concluded that mild to moderate hypothermia plays a significant role in cerebral protection after TBI. Several studies, including a Phase II clinical trial (Adelson, Ragheb, Muizelaar, Kaney, et al., 2005), have shown the potential of hypothermia for reducing ICP and managing intracranial hypertension in children. However, the effect on mortality and longer-term outcomes is much less clear-cut. A large-scale multi-center clinical trial in Canada showed that hypothermia did not improve the neurological outcome of children with TBI and could in fact increase the mortality rate (Hutchinson, Ward, Lacroix, Hébert, et al., 2008). More recently, a large, multi-center trial of hypothermia (the "Cool Kids Trial") was stopped for reasons of futility, after preliminary analyses showed a trend toward more negative outcomes for the hypothermia group.

The second edition of the US guidelines states that decompressive craniectomy can be considered in the management of severe TBI, based on a number of case series and small, controlled clinical trials that provided evidence that decompressive craniectomy can lead to reductions in mortality and better outcomes (Bell &

Kochanek, 2008). However, its beneficial effect has not been consistently demonstrated following pediatric TBI (Diedler, Sykora, Blatow, Juttler, et al., 2009). Research on decompressive craniectomy in adults with TBI has resulted in considerable controversy with the publication of the Decompressive Craniectomy (DECRA) study, which involved a large randomized clinical trial that resulted in poorer outcomes following craniectomy despite reductions in elevated ICP, fewer interventions for ICP, and fewer days in intensive care (Cooper, Rosenfeld, & Wolfe, 2012; Honeybul, Ho, Lind, & Gillett, 2011; Hossain-Ibrahim, Tanaris, & Wasserberg, 2012).

Medical interventions such as hypothermia and craniectomy provide an opportunity for multi-disciplinary research, in which medical staff and allied health professions can inform each other regarding the efficacy of the intervention on targeted outcome measures. Currently little evidence is available on long-term benefits and functional outcomes associated with such interventions in pediatric populations (Sivan, Neumann, Kent, Stroud, & Bhakta, 2010), and it is unlikely, given the specific characteristics of the developing brain, that adult interventions and associated evidence can be readily extrapolated to child TBI. Further research is clearly needed to determine the most effective interventions and whether multimodal therapy, which combines different approaches (e.g., hypothermia, hypertonic saline infusion, decompressive craniectomy), could enhance neuroprotection and result in better outcomes (Bell & Kochanek, 2008; Walker, Harting, Baumgartner, Fletcher, et al., 2009).

Guidelines for Mild TBI

The acute management of mild TBI, including concussion, initially reflects the same considerations that apply to more severe injuries. Once a primary survey of airway, cervical spine, breathing, and circulation is completed, an acute assessment of neurological status can occur (Grubenhoff & Provance, 2012). Often this involves the Glasgow Coma Scale, although other instruments may also come into play, such as the ChildSCAT3 (see Chapter 4 for more details on assessment methods and tools). The initial assessment will help determine whether the injury falls in the spectrum of mild TBI.

A critical decision in the acute management of concussion and mild TBI is whether to obtain a CT scan or any other type of neuroimaging. Because of concerns about the risks of cumulative exposure to radiation, particularly in the immature brain, routine CT scans of children with concussion or mild TBI are no longer considered acceptable. Substantial research has been devoted to developing decision rules for the use of CT scan in pediatric mild TBI. A variety of rules have been proposed, including the Children's Head Injury Algorithm for the Prediction of Important Clinical Events (CHALICE) from the United Kingdom (Dunning et al., 2006), the Canadian Assessment of Tomography for Childhood Head Injury (CATCH) rule (Osmond et al., 2010), and rules developed by the Pediatric Emergency Care

Applied Research Network (PECARN) in the United States (Kupperman et al., 2009). The rules have generally been developed to predict "clinically important brain injuries" or "significant intracranial injury," often defined as lesions necessitating neurosurgical intervention; notably, the PECARN rules were explicitly devised to predict which children were at low risk of such outcomes. The goal with decision rules is to develop a prognostic tool that has essentially no false negatives (i.e., 100% sensitivity) and as few false positives (i.e., high specificity) as possible. The rules typically incorporate information about mechanism of injury and acute signs and symptoms, as assessed through history and direct examination. Most of the rules have demonstrated negative predictive values approaching 100%, but positive predictive values are much lower, ranging from 2% to 8%, because of the low base rate of significant intracranial injuries among children with mild TBI.

Other neuroimaging techniques, including magnetic resonance imaging (MRI), are generally not used in the acute management of mild TBI. However, they may play a role in the assessment of risk for poor outcome or in clarifying the reasons for persistent problems. Ashwal, Tong, Bartnik-Olson, and Holshouser (2012) proposed an algorithm for the proposed use of neuroimaging in children with mild TBI that begins with a decision rule for CT scan but goes on to propose when MRI may be indicated. Further discussion of advanced neuroimaging techniques can be found in Chapter 5.

More general guidelines for the management of concussion and mild TBI have been published by a variety of organizations and authors (Lumba, Schnadower, & Joseph, 2011); for instance, the American Academy of Pediatrics and American Academy of Family Physicians (1999) offered some of the earliest guidelines for the management of mild TBI, and some hospitals have developed clinical pathways to guide clinical management (Kamerling, Lutz, Posner, & Vanore, 2003). More recent guidelines have been proposed specifically for managing sports concussion, by both the American Academy of Neurology (Giza, Kutcher, Ashwal, Barth, et al., 2013) and the American Academy of Pediatrics (Halstead & Walter, 2010). Among the key dispositional decisions that guidelines are meant to address is whether, after a concussion or mild TBI, an injured individual warrants hospitalization or is safe to be sent home. Large population–based studies suggest that children with isolated mild TBI who do not show sustained alterations in mental status, abnormal neurological findings, or abnormal CT findings do not require routine hospital admission (Adams, Frumiento, Shatney-Leach, & Vane, 2001; Holmes et al., 2011). Based in part on research of this sort, the rate of hospitalization for mild TBI has declined markedly over the last two decades in the United States and probably in other Western nations (Bowman, Bird, Aitken, & Tilford, 2008).

A target for current research is to provide an evidence base for clinical management of concussion and mild TBI in children and adolescents. At present, guidelines are inconsistent and have very little supporting data for decisions regarding return to play or return to sports. An example of a typical set of guidelines is illustrated in Table 9.1.

TABLE 9.1 Royal Children's Hospital Concussion Guidelines: Treatment and at Home Care

Rehabilitation stage	Exercise at each stage	Goal
1. No activity	Complete physical and mental rest.	Recovery
2. Light aerobic exercise	Walking, swimming, or stationary cycling. No resistance training.	Increase heart rate
3. Sport-specific exercise	Running drills in football (soccer or AFL), hockey, and other ball games. No head-impact activities.	Add movement
4. Non-contact training drills	Passing drills in football (soccer) and other ball games. May start progressive resistance training.	Exercise and coordination
5. Full-contact practice	Participate in normal training activities.	Restore confidence and assess function by coaching staff
6. Return to play	Normal game play.	

The majority of concussions will get better on their own over several days. To recover, the brain and body need to rest. Physical exercise and activities that require concentration (video or computer games, text messaging, schoolwork, etc.) may make symptoms worse and delay recovery. Children and adolescents with concussion need more time to recover than adults.

Use the steps in the table to safely return to playing sports.

Instructions

1. Each step takes at least 24 hours (a total of at least seven days).
2. Your child should move to the next step only if he or she has no concussion complaints.
3. If concussion complaints recur, go back to the previous step.
4. If your child cannot advance to the next step without concussion complaints, you should see your doctor before returning to playing sports.

FOLLOW UP

Talk to your doctor if you are unsure whether your child can progress to the next stage or can fully return to play. Go back to your doctor or hospital immediately if you are worried for any reason or if your child has any one of the following:

- Unusual or confused behavior
- Severe or persistent headache that is not relieved by paracetamol

- Frequent vomiting
- Bleeding or discharge from the ear or nose
- A fit or convulsion, or spasm of the face, arms, or legs
- Difficulty in waking up
- Difficulty in staying awake.

KEY POINTS TO REMEMBER

- The majority of concussions will get better on their own over several days.
- Follow the "return to play" steps carefully, ensuring at least 24 hours for each step.
- Talk to your doctor if you are unsure whether your child can progress to the next stage or can fully return to play.

Future Directions

Despite clear advances in the acute management of child TBI, the evidence base guiding clinical decisions remains scant. Over the next decade, research should result in a variety of advances in clinical care. For instance, research on biomarkers suggests that they provide an important tool in the diagnosis and prognosis of pediatric TBI. A variety of serum and CSF biomarkers, which include brain-specific proteins like S100β, markers of axonal injury like α–II spectrin, and inflammatory cytokines, have shown promise in discriminating TBI from other injuries, identifying intracranial injury in children with mild TBI, and assisting in outcome prediction following TBI (Berger & Zuckerbraun, 2012). Multiple methods can be used to screen for multiple markers simultaneously (Buttram et al., 2007).

Other advances in the management of child TBI are likely to involve more sophisticated neuromonitoring, including the measurement of partial pressure of oxygen (PbO$_2$). The measurement of PbO$_2$ may be relevant to assessing the effects of hyperventilation and to test for autoregulation within the brain, but it may be especially critical for assessing brain oxygenation and preventing hypoxia (Bell & Kochanek, 2008). The second edition of the *Guidelines for Medical Management of Severe Traumatic Brain Injury for Infants, Children, and Adolescents* (Kochanek et al., 2012) recommended thresholds for PbO$_2$ if it is monitored.

Methodological advances in research on treatment effectiveness may also lead to improvements in clinical care. In recent years, concern about the emphasis on randomized clinical trials for assessing treatment effectiveness has grown, not only because of the difficulties inherent in conducting such trials, but also because of their repeated failures in many contexts to advance treatment of TBI (Adelson, 2010). This concern has led to calls for more comparative effectiveness studies, which rely on natural variations in care across multiple sites and large numbers of patients to detect the effectiveness of specific interventions (Maas & Menon, 2012; Maas, Menon, Lingsma, Pineda, et al., 2012; Powell, Temkin, Machamer, & Dikmen, 2002). Several multidisciplinary, international studies of child TBI designed to take advantage of comparative effectiveness methodologies are underway.

10

EVIDENCE-BASED TREATMENT AND INTERVENTION APPROACHES

Introduction

TBI is associated with a threefold increase in cognitive, social, behavioral, and vocational difficulties worldwide (National Pediatric Trauma Registry, 1993). Incidence of TBI based on hospital admissions has been reported at between 100 and 300 per 100,000 per year for children and young adults, with 1 in 30 newborns suffering a TBI by age 16 (Cassidy et al., 2004; Crowe et al., 2009), with the most common type of TBI being a closed-head injury (Davis & Vogel, 1995). It has been estimated that one-third of children, post-TBI, would benefit from rehabilitation (Michaud, Rivara, Grady, & Reay, 1992) to prevent and/or minimize poor outcome and so improve quality of life. Despite this, limited availability of such resources has been reported, with few children offered rehabilitation/intervention (Cronin, 2001).

The aim of this chapter is to (a) provide an overview of approaches to rehabilitation/intervention following pediatric TBI; (b) present intervention research in the acute and longer-term post-TBI for children and adolescents; and (c) comment on the evaluation of studies in the area of intervention and the process for implementation into clinical care.

Management/Intervention: The Process Following Mild vs. Moderate to Severe TBI

Mild TBI

As discussed in more detail in Chapter 7, following a mild TBI children and adolescents may present with confusion, disorientation, fatigue, and a brief period of altered consciousness—"post-concussional syndrome" (PCS). Though cognitive difficulties may be evident in areas such as attention and speed of processing (Beers, 1992; Boll, 1983), there is controversy regarding long-term uneventful recovery (Asarnow et al., 1995) and persisting longer-term cognitive and/or psychological difficulties (McKinlay et al., 2002; McKinlay, 2009). In adults, PCS commonly persists for only several days; in children and adolescents, the recovery path is more prolonged, with most victims demonstrating PCS for up to 30 days and longer (Barlow et al., 2010; Yeates et al., 2012), with 5–10% remaining symptomatic at one year (Barlow et al., 2010; Olsson et al., 2013). Though some young people adjust to these limitations, a significant number will have difficulty adjusting and will develop depression, anxiety and post-traumatic stress, and poor quality of life (Anderson, Brown, et al., 2011; Max et al., 2011).

There is also controversy regarding return to play (in a sports context) and return to school decision rules, leaving guidelines for intervention lacking a strong evidence base. The Consensus Statements on concussion in sport (Aubry, Cantu, Dvorak, Graf-Baumann, et al., 2002; McCrory et al., 2004, 2009, 2013) have attempted to provide guidelines for return to play, with a graduated return to play protocol (see Table 10.1). However, it has been suggested that these management recommendations could be applied down to the age of 13 years, with younger children requiring different assessment tools that are developmentally sensitive, with inclusion of patient, parent, teacher, and school input. The panel also agreed that no return to sport or activity should occur before successful return to school, with no return to play until the child is completely symptom free. However, decisions continue to remain in the clinical judgment of a multidisciplinary team and depend on the circumstances specific to each individual case.

TABLE 10.1 Return to Play Rules Post-Concussion Guidelines

Rehabilitation stage	Exercises	Objective
No activity	Physical/cognitive rest	Recovery
Light aerobic exercise	Keep intensity < 70% permitted heart rate—e.g., walking, swimming; no resistance training	Increase heart rate
Sport-specific exercise	No head-impact activities— e.g., running drills in soccer	Add movement
Non-contact training drills	More complex training drills—e.g., passing drills in football; start resistance training	Exercise, coordination, training load
Full contact practice	Normal training activities once given medical clearance	Skills assessed by coaching staff
Return to play	Normal play	

Source: Adapted from McCrory et al. (2013).

Therefore, as mentioned in previous chapters, following a mild TBI a child is seen in the emergency department and monitored for a period of time to ensure that symptoms do not escalate. If no further monitoring or treatment is required, the child is discharged home, with advice regarding common symptoms of concussion and return to play and school.

Moderate to Severe TBI

Following a significant TBI, in which complications (e.g., edema) are developing as the child/adolescent is transported to hospital, the pattern is quite different. In these more severe cases, cognitive problems are common, with long-term support necessary, particularly at developmental transition stages (e.g., completion of primary school, entry into high school and tertiary studies, entering the workforce), where skills expected to emerge may be delayed and/or deficient (Anderson & Catroppa, 2006).

Behavioral Management in Post-Traumatic Amnesia

While the child is in coma, intervention is commenced, provided the child is medically stable, and is initially focused on sensory stimulation. Once the child emerges from coma, basic functions such as feeding and physical strength are evaluated. During this time, children may present with restlessness and agitation and may also be experiencing post-traumatic amnesia (PTA; Anderson & Catroppa, 2006). During PTA, confusion, disorientation, and loss of memory of recent events (High, Levin, & Gary, 1989) are also common. Because agitation, restlessness, and disorientation can place individuals at risk and limit their progress in rehabilitation therapy (Lequerica, Rapport, Loeher, Axelrod, et al., 2007), management strategies are essential at this point in recovery.

Allied Health Team Involvement

Once the child is relatively stable, the whole allied health team is involved. In the early days following the injury, the team assesses the child's current level of function, identifying specific impairments that will affect his or her activity and participation. The team also works with the family to help them understand how the child is functioning now, as well as how they can help in the recovery process. At this point, there is also nursing and medical input. The nurse coordinates the patient's management and acts as the link between medical, nursing, and allied health teams. Though the allied team works together, each discipline has a role in which they assess particular outcomes—for example, the speech therapist will assess speech and language, the occupational therapist will assess motor skills, the neuropsychologist will be involved regarding issues of PTA and will investigate cognitive outcomes such as attention and memory, the social worker may discuss issues with family members, and a clinical psychologist may work with the child regarding adjustment issues. Educational consultants are also involved at the inpatient stage, often with a number of roles, which may include contacting the school to inform them of the child's condition and to obtain information regarding premorbid function and, when needed, assisting the child with actual schoolwork.

This allied health team will come together during team meetings and case conferences to discuss key goals and priorities and to coordinate timetables to allow focus on specific goals (e.g., clearing a morning schedule to prioritize a self-care routine). While rehabilitation is provided for the child, education and support are provided for the family.

Discharge

Prior to discharge, children with more severe injury are allowed to go on day, overnight, or weekend leave to give them a chance to go home for a short time, but also to give the team an idea of how they cope at home. This provides an opportunity for the physical therapist and occupational therapist to see the child at home and, if necessary, to make modifications to the house to suit the child's needs.

The timing of discharge of the child from hospital is decided by the allied health team. The decision is based on a number of factors, which include the child's level of function, the child's post-discharge environment, the family's adjustment and their ability to cope, the capacity of local services to provide ongoing therapy at a level that is appropriate to the child's needs, and the decision on whether the child would benefit more from being at home than having daily therapy as an inpatient. Once discharge is decided upon, it is planned via inpatient meeting discussions of staff, via meetings with the family, and with the coordination of local services and therapy teams. Contact is also made with the child's school early on in rehabilitation, and at time of discharge a handover meeting is held in which information and discharge reports are discussed with the school staff. A return to school plan is articulated, and teleconferences and school visits follow as necessary. For children who remain with the team for rehabilitation as outpatients, more communication with their school is planned, in which key school staff are invited to attend brain injury "education" meetings, while also allowing for the sharing of ideas and information about the particular child. Successful re-integration into society relies on the coordination of home/family, school, and medical/allied health care (Semrud-Clikeman, 2010), with supports provided as needed for the child, family, and other integral services (Byard, Fine, & Reed, 2011).

Rehabilitation as a Collaborative Process

As is evident by the information provided regarding the process of inpatient rehabilitation, it is clear that therapists do not work in isolated discipline-specific areas, but in fact work as a team, sharing the responsibility of care for a particular child.

Furthermore, the multidisciplinary team, while heading the rehabilitation process, is now incorporating the child (where applicable) and the family in the decision-making process and in the identification of goals considered most important to meet the needs of the child and the family. There has been a focus on identifying the needs of the child and family in order to indicate where goals need to be targeted. This collaborative model of a multidisciplinary team and the family and child, with the discussion of specific goals to be targeted, has become known as the "goal attainment model."

Recently, a number of researchers have evaluated such programs in order to provide an evidence base for their use in rehabilitation settings. Cusick, McIntyre, Novack, Lannin, and Lowe (2006) reported that the active involvement of parents throughout the process of setting and implementing goals increased their feeling of competence and that goals based on families' preferences and concerns encouraged the family to pursue the specified and agreed-upon goal. A recent paper (An & Palisano, 2013) considered a four-step process of collaboration, involving (1) mutually agreed-upon goals, (2) shared planning, (3) shared implementation, and (4) shared evaluation. It was concluded that the model may have utility for optimizing collaboration between families and professionals—that it may foster family empowerment and therefore optimize outcomes for the child and family. In general, results from collaborative goal setting have been reported to be of benefit in promoting better outcomes for child and family, with results concluding that there should therefore be investment of resources to make it an integral part of the rehabilitation process (Brewer, Pollock, & Wright, 2013).

Intervention in the acute stage. Pharmacological intervention may be implemented in order to manage agitation and restlessness as seen during PTA (Mysiw & Sandel, 1997). Such agents may include carbamazepine, antidepressants, methylphenidate, and amantadine; however, due to the lack of well-controlled clinical trials, no drug has yet been approved for the management of PTA. Furthermore, agitation may not have a single underlying neuropathologic mechanism, and therefore individuals may respond differently to the same drug, with a further complexity being the possibility of side effects from the drugs (Mysiw & Sandel, 1997). While reducing aggression, drugs may also worsen problems in cognitive areas, such as arousal, attention, and motor control (Flanagan, 2009). Though there appears to be a role for pharmacological intervention, there is limited evidence to guide clinicians in this area, with some researchers advocating for the combination of pharmacological and non-pharmacological approaches (Flanagan, 2009; Levy, Berson, Cook, Bollegala, et al., 2005).

Further management suggestions in the adult literature for disorientation and agitation have included minimizing unexpected situational changes, providing an organized and structured environment, and the implementation of music therapy. Music therapy has been implemented with an adult population post-injury, and it was found that when listening to either familiar recorded or live music, clear improvements in orientation and a reduction in agitation were evident (Baker,

2001). This study demonstrated that music therapy did not overstimulate the individual and was a viable method of managing the individual in PTA. Bower et al., (2010), using a mixed-methods case study, investigated the efficacy of music therapy for a child with significant cognitive impairment and reduced level of consciousness following severe TBI and experiencing agitation during PTA. Data collection took place for the first 10 days of PTA (video recorded pre-, during, and post-music therapy). Inconclusive results were reported with regard to the effect of music therapy in reducing agitation in this severe case. However, it was found that the music therapy offered an environment in which the participant was able to maximize her periods of awareness and thus was able to optimize early recovery of consciousness and cognitive abilities. This case demonstrated that even in the severest of cases, music therapy can play a role in recovery, with its potential in less impaired participants still to be researched.

Interventions in the Longer-Term Post-Injury

In the months and years following injury, direct, indirect, medical, family, and community approaches to intervention are considered in order to facilitate recovery and improve long-term outcome. Interventions in the longer-term post-discharge and the years following the injury are difficult to develop and implement. Randomized controlled trials do not often suit cognitive and behavioral interventions; therefore there is a need for alternative models to determine feasibility and efficacy. Often, participation in interventions requires a considerable time commitment and places a burden on families, particularly those that are not geographically close to health centers. Therefore, there is a need for different approaches across ages and time post-injury, with a focus on key outcome measures that will capture the efficacy of the intervention program with regard to everyday functioning (Penkman, 2004).

A variety of intervention approaches have been implemented in research protocols (Bryck & Fisher, 2012). The limited research studies in this area will now be presented, in order to demonstrate how these approaches have been incorporated into research designs and that there is a clear need for the evaluation of these studies in order to build an evidence base to support their implementation into clinical care (Kneafsey & Gawthorpe, 2004).

(i) Direct Approach

With such an approach, the focus is on the cognitive impairment that has been identified. The child/adolescent is then trained, via specific exercises, in an attempt to retrain, stimulate, and so improve skills in these areas (Rothi & Horner, 1983). In the adult area, it has been reported that direct approaches may be more effective in specific domains, such as attention (Gray, Robertson, Pentland, & Anderson, 1992; Mateer, Kerns, & Eso, 2006). In the child domain, it has also been used to improve skills in attention, executive skills, and memory (Brett & Laatsch, 1998; Glang, Singer, Cooley, & Tish, 1992; Lawson & Rice, 1989; Suzman, Morris, Morris, & Milan, 1997; Thomson, 1995). However, there is limited evidence to support its effectiveness and/or generalization to daily functions (Park & Ingles, 2001; Wood, 1987).

(ii) Indirect Approaches

Behavioral Compensation

When using this approach, individuals are taught to perform various activities and tasks using alternative strategies and so are compensating for cognitive deficits. The aim is to reduce the functional impact of the impairment and attain goal behaviors (Stuss, Mateer, & Sohlberg, 1994). This approach suggests that compensatory approaches, rather than cognitive retraining, will lead to improved performance (Park & Ingles, 2001).

Behavior Modification Strategies

Strategies in this area include the use of behavioral interventions. These may include positive and negative reinforcement, modeling, and role-playing (Burke, Wesolowski, & Guth, 1988); the implementation of token economies (Mottram & Berger-Gross, 2004); the writing of behavioral contracts, the use of peer facilitators (Kazdin, 1984); saturated cues (Crowley & Miles, 1991); and graphic advance organizers and "goal-plan-do-review" (Feeney & Ylvisaker, 2003). These trained behaviors are measured directly at the same time that treatment is given (Ponsford, Sloan, & Snow, 1995), and therefore one can evaluate whether the target behavior has changed due to the intervention.

Environmental Modifications and Supports

This requires a collaborative approach, including the family, school, and broader community. Applications may include the simplification of tasks, allowing the child more time to complete tasks, the reduction of noise, the removal of other potential distractions (Mateer, 1999), and the use of external aids or cues, such as lists, diaries, alarms, or paging systems. Often, the emphasis of pediatric rehabilitation is on modifying the child's environment in order to promote best level of function.

Psycho-Educational Approaches

Education targeted to the child has shown less promising results (Beardmore, Tate, & Liddle, 1999) when compared with an adolescent/young adult group (Catroppa, Anderson, & Muscara, 2009) and a parent sample (Ponsford et al., 2001), where both latter groups were shown to benefit. It is also essential that information regarding possible short-term difficulties and longer-term deficits, and how these may limit the child's ability to cope with routine expectations and interfere with quality of life, be provided at the level of the child's school and community (Anderson, 2003).

Psychological Treatments

There has been little investigation of approaches to emotional, social, and behavioral issues in the pediatric field (Ylvisaker et al., 2005). Methods employed with children have included behavioral methods, psychotherapy, pharmacological approaches, and medical approaches (Clifton, 2004; Mahalick, Carmel, Greenbert, Molofsky, et al., 1998; Napolitano, Elovic, & Qureshi, 2005). In an adult study (Hodgson, McDonald, Tate, & Gertier, 2005) post-intervention improvement in behavior was reported following cognitive behavior therapy (CBT) for social anxiety post-TBI. Work in our laboratory is now underway in adapting and implementing a CBT program for adolescents, post-TBI, who are presenting with anxiety (Soo et al., project in progress).

Psychostimulants

Though no medications have yet been found that meet a practice standard for the treatment of cognitive impairments in a population with TBI (Cicerone, Levin, Malec, Stuss, & Whyte, 2006), medications that modulate neurochemical systems have been reported to have possible treatment potential (McDowell, Whyte, & D'Esposito, 1997). In some cases, pharmacological approaches may be employed to alleviate both acute and more chronic symptoms, such as attention deficits post-TBI (Morris, Forsyth, Parslow, Tasker, & Hawley, 2006). However, though pharmacological management of neurobehavioral sequelae is common, the evidence to guide this practice is sparse, with a need for combination therapy, rather than reliance on a single agent, and the identification of specific subpopulations that may benefit (Chew & Zafonte, 2009; Walker et al., 2009).

Family-Based Interventions

The benefits of including significant others has been shown in the recovery process (Bedell, Cohn, & Dumas, 2005; Braga, Da Paz Junior, & Ylvisaker, 2005; Feeney & Ylvisaker, 2003; Mottram & Berger-Gross, 2004; Wade et al., 2006a; Ylvisaker et al., 2001) as an alternative, or in addition, to a clinician-delivered approach (Braga et al., 2005), while also using avenues, such as Internet-based, interactive multimedia modalities (Glang, McLaughlin, & Schroeder, 2007; Wade et al., 2005) and face-to-face or telephone intervention (Woods et al., 2014).

TABLE 10.2 Types and Timing of Intervention

Timing	Intervention
Coma	Sensory stimulation
Acute medical	Hypothermia
	Craniotomy
	Medications/psychostimulants
PTA	Commencement of basic intervention for difficulties in cognition, speech and mobility
	Music therapy
Post-PTA	Continued inpatient intervention for difficulties in cognition, speech, behavior and mobility
Outpatient therapy	Intervention to assist re-entry into home and school:
	Direct approach
	Behavioral compensation
	Behavior modification strategies
	Environmental modification and supports
	Psycho-educational approaches
	Psychological treatments
	Intervention at times of transition
	Family-based
	School-based
	Community-based
	Vocational

Source: Adapted from Catroppa & Anderson (2010).

Though the above approaches to intervention have been introduced (see Table 10.2), studies incorporating such approaches to prevent or reduce difficulties following pediatric TBI are few. The following section will present such intervention research in the pediatric field.

Intervention Research for Cognitive Difficulties

(Refer to Table 10.3 for common interventions for specific outcomes.)

(I) Executive Functioning (EF) and Attentional Functioning

When investigating difficulties in the areas of EF and attention (Anderson, 2002; Mirsky et al., 1991), a number of general intervention strategies have been put forth by Dawson and Guare (2004) and Ylvisaker and Feeney (2002), with the goal of implementing such strategies into the classroom setting. These authors suggest a number of possible general intervention strategies; however, it is outside the scope of this chapter to discuss these in detail, and so for a comprehensive review refer

TABLE 10.3 Summary of Common Intervention Approaches for Specific Outcome/Areas perhaps this table would be better placed after the vocational section

Outcome/area	Intervention Method
Cognitive	Direct approach
	Behavioral compensation
	Behavior modification strategies
	Environmental modifications and supports
	Psycho-educational approach
	Psychological treatments
Social/behavioral	Behavioral compensation
	Behavior modification techniques
	Psychological treatments
Psychiatric/emotional	Environmental modifications and supports
	Psychological treatments
	Pharmacological
Motor	Direct approach
	Environmental modifications and supports
Family	Psycho-educational approach
	Behavior modification techniques
	Cognitive behavior therapy
School	Psycho-educational approach
Community	Psycho-educational approach
Vocational	Psycho-educational approach
	Environmental modifications and supports

Source: Adapted from Catroppa & Anderson (2008).

to Dawson and Guare (2004); Slifer and Amari (2009); Ylvisaker (1985); Ylvisaker and Feeney (2002); and Ylvisaker, Szekeres, and Feeney (1998).

In a study by Burke et al. (1988), an intervention was implemented to improve attention and concentration, memory, problem-solving skills, and social judgment in a group of five adolescents severely injured in motor vehicle accidents. With regard to attention and concentration, self-control and antecedent control strategies were implemented. In order to improve self-regulation, intervention included self-instructional training, modeling, role-playing, reinforcement, and group feedback. The intervention was considered successful, as four out of five adolescents returned home to live with their parents and were able to return to public schools.

Also interested in improving attention and concentration, Brett and Laatsch (1998) trained teachers to administer rehabilitation tasks via the use of a computer and flashcards. Minimal improvement was seen, and so the intervention was considered unsuccessful, with inconsistent findings often evident (Robertson, 1990) when relying on computer-based intervention. Attention Process Training (APT) was also tried using both a single-case methodology and a group approach

(Thomson, 1995; Thomson & Kerns, 2000), and though some participants showed improvement, strong support was not shown for the use of APT.

Using a combination of process-specific and metacognitive strategies for the remediation of attention, Galbiati et al. (2009) investigated 65 patients post-TBI between the ages of 6–18 years. It was found that using this combined approach of six months' duration, results showed significantly improved attention performance on standardized measures, as well as some improvement in the adaptive area.

Implementing rehabilitation at 18 months following severe injury, Crowley and Miles (1991) reported on an adolescent case study. The participant was a 16-year-old male presenting with difficulties with applying himself to a task and then self-monitoring his progress. A behaviorally based intervention was implemented over 40 one-hour sessions via the use of saturated cues and by charting progress. The outcome measure was performance on an algebra review test and completion of homework, and results suggested some improvement in these areas. Selznick and Savage (2000) also implemented a behaviorally based intervention with three adolescent boys presenting with self-monitoring problems post-injury. The outcome measures focused on task behavior, accuracy, and productivity. The intervention, a behavioral compensation approach (e.g., the use of cues), improved self-monitoring, which in turn led to gains in accuracy and productivity. Of importance, generalization was also evident when the intervention was withdrawn and gains were still evident.

In a study with broader outcome measures, including memory, attention, planning, and organizational problems, a sample of 143 subjects, following brain injury and ranging in age from 8–83 years, took part in an intervention program (Wilson, Emslie, Quirk, & Evans, 2001). The intervention constituted a radio-paging system where reminders were transmitted to each individual on his or her pager, and it was found to improve everyday problems of memory and planning. However, the broad age range made its applicability to children unclear. Addressing attentional difficulties only, Luton, Reed-Knight, Loiselle, O'Toole, and Blount (2011) found that a shortened version of the Cognitive Rehabilitation Program (CRP) showed promise as a brief treatment for neurocognitive deficits.

Case studies were reported for three severely injured children aged from 6 to 10 years (Glang et al., 1992). The intervention was reliant upon behavioral principles, including task analysis, modeling, and shaping, with the goal of improvement in problem-solving strategies and related skills. The intervention was found to be successful in areas such as self-monitoring and mathematics. Similarly, Suzman et al. (1997) investigated five children between the ages of 6 and 11 years who had sustained severe head injuries six to nine months previously. These children also presented with problem-solving difficulties and were offered a complex intervention consisting of metacognitive training, self-instructional training, self-regulation training, attribution training, and reinforcement. A computerized problem-solving task (*Think Quick,* 1987), as well as parent and teacher measures, were used to evaluate the intervention program. Results revealed substantial improvement on both trained tasks and some standardized tests of problem-solving.

Using a psychostimulant approach, Bakker and Waugh (2000) described the case of a 7-year-old boy with a history of aquired brain injury (ABI) who underwent a trial of stimulant medication for the management of attentional problems. Implementing one-week treatment for each of dexamphetamine and methylphenidate, and two weeks of placebo, a double-blind placebo-controlled trial was conducted. No definite support for the efficacy of the stimulants was reported, but the researchers felt that such an approach has potential in individual cases. In contrast, others have reported results from a double-blind, placebo-controlled, cross-over experimental design, suggesting that psychostimulants are an effective agent in the treatment of such attentional deficits following child TBI (Mahalick et al., 1998).

More recently, a pilot intervention program (case design) based on a psychoeducational approach was implemented with three adolescents/young adults (Catroppa, Anderson, & Muscara, 2009) with the goal of improving executive functioning skills. Findings from this series of case studies showed little benefit of intervention on standardized measures of EF, with no consistent improvements from pre- to post-intervention. In contrast, some changes were evident on functional measures for two of the three cases, suggesting that the content and delivery of the intervention may be efficacious at the level of day-to-day function. Another intervention pilot program (Catroppa et al., 2014), concerned with remediating attention and memory deficits, aimed to pilot the feasibility and efficacy of the English version of the Amsterdam Memory and Attention Training for Children (AMAT-C) and to identify ecologically valid measures sensitive to post-evaluation improvements. Results indicated improved performance in the areas of attention and memory from pre- to post-intervention, with gains maintained at six months post-intervention.

(ii) Memory

Vakil, Blachstein, Rochberg, and Vardi (2004) reported that children who sustained a TBI had difficulty transferring information into long-term storage, reflecting an inefficient learning strategy, which also implicated working memory (ability to manipulate the information held in memory) on tasks of an executive nature. Though intervention techniques for "memory" difficulties have been researched in adults: memory book training (Sohlberg & Mateer, 1989); notebook training (Schmitter-Edgecombe, Fahy, Whelan, & Long, 1995); use of compensatory devices and environmental modifications (Stringer, 2011; Wilson, 1996); and errorless learning (Wilson, Baddeley, & Evans, 1994), in comparison, little work has been implemented in the development and piloting of intervention techniques for a pediatric population.

Oberg and Turkstra (1998) intervened by employing an elaborative encoding paradigm with two severely injured adolescents and demonstrated improvements on the trained task. Using a direct approach, Lawson and Rice (1989) demonstrated improved list-learning ability. External cueing, via the use of a computerized reminder intervention program (*Neuropage*) improved memory and recall in children as young as 8 years of age (Wilson et al., 2001). Errorless learning was also compared to trial-and-error learning for declarative facts in a group of children who had sustained a TBI and met criteria for memory impairment (Landis, Hanten, Levin, Li, et al., 2006). Results did not support errorless learning as a generalized intervention for memory and learning problems, nor did it identify specific injury severity or age groups for which it would be efficacious to use errorless learning.

With a developmental perspective in mind, Wright and Limond (2004) described implicit (e.g., walking) and explicit (e.g., piece of knowledge) memory, with the latter including working memory. These authors suggested that younger children would benefit from the use of passive rehabilitation, including the use of environmental support, whereas older children would benefit instead from strategic intervention or assistance in improving the organization of material in memory. Considering event-based prospective memory impairments, McCauley et al. (2011) found that though monetary incentives improved memory at three months post-injury for children with moderate injury, it was not effective for those with severe injury.

In a recent randomized controlled trial conducted in Sweden, a weekly training intervention program was implemented (Van't Hooft et al., 2005, 2007) to improve children's attention and memory skills. Results showed improvements in neuropsychological measures of attention and memory post-intervention for the treatment group on standardized measures of outcome, with pilot data suggesting improved social relations and reduced parental stress. Another research team (Madsen-Sjo, Spellerberg, Weidner, & Kihlgren, 2010) also piloted this same intervention using a Danish version and integrated the intervention into the child's school. Though the sample size was small, significant improvement was reported in tests of learning and memory, but no change was seen in executive function.

Lajiness-O'Neill, Erdodi, and Bigler (2010) reviewed and examined moderators of outcome for memory and learning difficulties. These authors concluded that investigation of the efficacy of interventions for such difficulties was lacking, even though memory and learning difficulties are common post-injury. They reported that best practice includes systematic instructional methods in a context-sensitive approach, treatment with a basis in everyday life, and opportunities for maintenance and generalization of skills.

Intervention Research for Social/Behavioral Difficulties

Social and behavioral difficulties are often present following brain injury, and they can make re-integration into "everyday life" challenging. Intervention strategies in this area may include behavioral strategies, such as reinforcement, shaping, modeling, cuing, use of contracts, self-monitoring, anxiety-managing strategies, relaxation techniques, didactic class activities, and use of peer models (Dykeman, 2003). However, there is minimal research investigating these techniques with children.

Feeney and Ylvisaker (2003) investigated the effects of a cognitive behavioral intervention program on two severely injured young children who presented with challenging behavior, as well as organization and planning problems in the classroom. The intervention focused on (i) daily routine; (ii) positive momentum; (iii) reduction of errors; (iv) escape communication; (v) adult communication style; (vi) graphic advance organizers; and (vii) "goal-plan-do-review" routine, with staff trained in a number of these areas. At the conclusion of the program, challenging behaviors had significantly decreased in intensity and frequency, with maintenance of skills evident in the longer term. Similarly, Mottram and Berger-Gross (2004) evaluated a behavioral intervention program (e.g., program rules, token economy) for three children with brain injury aged 8–14 years. The methodology employed was a multiple baseline design across individuals. Disruptive behavior was seen to decrease by 69% during the intervention phase, with maintenance at follow-up.

Slifer and Amari (2009) have recommended guidelines for behavior management post-TBI, and these include (i) direct behavioral observations, (ii) assessment of the environment, (iii) assessment of patient variables, and (iv) differential reinforcement of target behavior, so as to increase the preferred behavior and decrease disruptive behavior. Such a complex intervention would require monitoring and guidance by a trained behavioral psychologist/therapist.

In our laboratory, the "Signposts for Building Better Behaviour" program (Gavidia-Payne & Hudson, 2002; Hudson, Matthews, Gavidia-Payne, Cameron, et al., 2003), which has proven successful with families of children with intellectual and developmental difficulties, has been modified and adapted for a pediatric TBI population (Woods, Catroppa, Giallo, Matthews, & Anderson, 2012). Post-TBI, children may be at significant risk of serious behavioral and social difficulties. Therefore the program, based on a cognitive-behavioral approach, aims to provide support and teach strategies to families of children with acquired brain injury in order to prevent and reduce challenging behaviors (e.g., disruptive behavior, poor social skills). Forty-eight parents of children aged between 3 to 12 years with mild, moderate, and severe injuries received the intervention in face-to-face ($n = 23$) or telephone-support ($n = 25$) format. All parents approved of the skills taught and a majority felt the materials were helpful in both managing behavior and teaching new skills. The program was reported to both reduce the number of challenging behaviors in injured children and lower parental stress and family burden (Woods et al., 2014).

Intervention for Psychiatric/Emotional Functioning

Intervention for psychiatric and emotional functioning may be approached clinically with the inclusion of counseling, psychology, or psychiatry services, often using a cognitive-behavioral approach (Noggle & Pierson, 2010) or the use of medications (Mahalick et al., 1998; Napolitano et al., 2005).

Gagnon, Galli, Friedman, Grilli, and Iverson (2009) reported on an alternative intervention for the management of children slower to recover after a sport-related concussion. The goal was to reduce the chance of symptoms becoming chronic in areas including stress, mild depression, anxiety, anger, loneliness, and diminished vigor. The exercise-based intervention was administered at one month post-injury. For those who participated, a rapid recovery was seen, with return to normal lifestyles and sports participation.

An area now receiving attention in alleviating symptoms of emotional regulation, including depressive symptoms, is that of Positive Psychology interventions. In a recent meta-analysis that included both adult and child/adolescent studies, and concerned with the alleviation of depressive symptoms, it was found that these interventions do reduce depressive symptoms and enhance well-being (Sin & Lyubomirsky, 2009).

As mentioned earlier, in our laboratory an intervention is in progress with the goal of adapting and trying a cognitive behavioral therapy (CBT) program for managing anxiety (Soo et al., study in progress), which is based on a program currently available for youth without brain injury (Rapee, Lyneham, Schniering, Wuthrish, et al., 2006). This adapted program is now complete, and it includes a revised manual to allow use by health professionals working with this population. An RCT has recently commenced.

Psychopharmacological methods may also be used to manage psychiatric and emotional functioning. In a review combining pediatric and adult samples (Whyte, Vaccaro, Grieb-Neff, & Hart, 2002), three specific drugs were investigated: methylphenidate, amphetamine, and dextroamphetamine. The positive effect of methylphenidate was reported on at least one outcome measure in the area of mood/behavior, whereas dextroamphetamine results were inconsistent. Beers, Skold, Dixon, & Adelson (2005) investigated the efficacy and safety of a dopamine agonist, amantadine hydrochloride (AMH), in the treatment of neurobehavioral sequelae following pediatric TBI, with parents reporting an improvement in behavior. Williams (2007) reviewed the amantadine literature (five studies) and found that behavioral and cognitive outcome measures yielded mixed results.

Intervention for Motor/Physical Difficulties

Post-injury children may be in need of physical therapy (PT) interventions to improve mobility in affected limbs. Dumas, Haley, Carey, and Shen (2004) reported that therapeutic exercise was the most frequently reported intervention. It was found that, though the correspondence was small, intensity (as measured by the length of stay in the rehabilitation unit) of PT intervention in an inpatient rehabilitation hospital was related to improved functional mobility, suggesting the need for the opportunity of repetition of the trained skill.

In a review by Holden (2005), virtual reality (VR) environments for motor rehabilitations were discussed, as well as the applicability of such an intervention for those with acquired brain injury and other clinical groups requiring an enhancement in motor skills. Overall, VR was reported to be advantageous in supporting and enhancing learning by the provision of repetition, feedback, and motivation, all considered important elements in motor learning. Furthermore, four major findings emerged from this review: (i) patients appear capable of learning with a VR environment; (ii) movements taught and learned in VR transferred to real work-equivalent tasks and also to untrained tasks; (iii) some advantages of VR training over training in a "real" environment are evident; and (iv) VR has not resulted in reports of cybersickness (Holden, 2005).

In a recent review (Galvin, McDonald, Catroppa, & Anderson, 2011), VR was again seen as an emerging area of clinical and research practice following pediatric neurological impairment. The review was concerned with current evidence for use of VR interventions to improve upper-limb function of children with neurological impairment. Five studies (one RCT and four case studies) were found and critiqued, with studies reported to have methodological limitations that limit generalizability. These results suggest that, though VR appears promising in the retraining of upper-limb function, research in this area is currently at an emerging stage, with further studies required to evaluate this intervention strategy.

Though in the last decade neuropsychological VR applications are emerging both for improvement of motor and other impairments, as seen by the cited review articles, the use of VR in a pediatric population following brain injury is yet to emerge (Penn, Rose, & Johnson, 2009). In our laboratory, we have an intervention program in progress using VR, aimed at improving upper-limb function of children that have an acquired brain injury (Galvin et al., study in progress). Children have been allocated to the treatment group or to standard clinical care, with a control group also recruited. This study is unique in this area and will clarify the role of VR in the improvement of mobility post-injury.

Interventions: Family-/School Based-/Community-Based—The Role of Educating Caregivers

The important role of caregivers, including families, teachers, and the community, in the recovery process following brain injury has been highlighted (Feeney & Ylvisaker, 2003; Kreutzer, Stejskal, Ketchum, Matwitz, et al., 2009; Mottrom & Berger-Gross, 2004; Ylvisaker et al., 2001). Therefore, an intervention program may incorporate the education of caregivers (including the injured child/adolescent if appropriate) with regard to the mechanisms of the injury, possible short-and long-term consequences of the injury, the recovery process, and the role of intervention in both prevention and dealing with residual impairments.

Family-Based Intervention

When introduced with an information session regarding brain injury (Beardmore et al., 1999), it was demonstrated that parents did appear to show improved understanding of their child's difficulty following a single session. Ponsford et al. (2001)

evaluated a group of children who had sustained a mild brain injury and compared them to children with minor injuries not involving the head. One group of children who had sustained a mild ABI were seen one week post-injury, and the family was provided with a booklet outlining common symptoms and suggested coping strategies. Another group was not given the booklet and was reviewed at three months post-injury. Results indicated that the latter group generally reported more symptoms and was more stressed three months after the injury. The provision of the booklet appeared to lower the incidence of ongoing problems by reducing anxiety.

Braga and colleagues (2005) explored the effectiveness of a clinician-delivered versus a family-supported intervention. Both groups showed improvement, but only those with family support demonstrated significant improvements in physical and cognitive domains. Similarly, Arco and Bishop (2009) reported on a number of case studies where parents were trained to use positive behavior support in the home. Parents, with the assistance of the health professional, participated in observations and assessment of their child's behavior problems and in the planning and implementation of the intervention. Results suggested that this parent-implemented approach was effective.

The methodology of a few family-based projects has focused on the training of parents/family to improve the outcome of an implemented intervention. As mentioned earlier, the Signposts program is family based—the parents are trained in strategies to manage challenging behavior in their child, with results showing promise in reducing such behaviors and improving family functioning (Woods et al., 2014). Glang, McLaughlin, and Schroeder (2007) trained parents of children with brain injury in educational advocacy skills, using an interactive multimedia intervention. Parents in the treatment group scored higher in the areas of application, knowledge, and attitudes in comparison to the control group.

Using web-based technology, (Antonini, Raj, Oberjohn, & Wade, 2012; Wade et al., 2005, 2009; Wade, Walz, et al., 2011) the feasibility and efficacy of a web-based family intervention addressing problem-solving skills for children and adolescents post-injury was examined, with results suggesting it would be a promising intervention tool. Wade, Carey, and Wolfe (2006a, 2006b) further investigated the efficacy of this problem-solving family intervention and reported that it held promise for reducing child behavior and adjustment problems post-TBI. With regard to adolescent findings (Wade, Chertkoff Walz, et al., 2008), significant improvements were found in parent-reported adolescent internalizing behaviors, self-reported adolescent depressive symptoms, parental depression, and parent-adolescent conflict, providing preliminary evidence for the efficacy of this approach with an older age group. With a focus on parental outcome, this web-based intervention was also found to reduce stress, anxiety, and depressive symptoms and facilitate parental adaptation in families of children with moderate to severe TBI (Wade et al., 2006a).

Cole, Paulos, Cole, and Tankard (2009) published a review of family intervention guidelines for pediatric acquired brain injuries. General findings identified psychological distress in carers and siblings of a child following brain injury and that family functioning also affected the injured child's recovery. The guidelines were put forth to inform those implementing interventions at a family level and included (i) the selection of developmentally appropriate interventions; (ii) a match between the intervention and the family; (iii) provision of advocacy and injury education; (iv) a focus on family realignment; (v) an adjustment of the child's environment; and (vi) the provision of skills training to the child and the family. As family-based intervention studies are few, these guidelines were described as theoretically derived, requiring more research evidence to support their efficacy.

School-Based Intervention

Clinical experience has indicated that, at both the school and community level, those dealing with a child or adolescent following traumatic brain injury need to be provided with information regarding the child's recovery patterns; the possible long-term deficits in cognitive, behavioral, and social areas; and how these difficulties may limit the child's ability to cope in these settings (Anderson, 2003).

In a study by Gfoerer, Wade, and Wu (2008), results indicated that few school-based supports were perceived for children post-injury, but the greatest unmet need was in the area of behavioral and emotional support. This paper highlighted the importance of intervention at times of transition and the need for communication between the school setting and other agencies in order to ensure smooth reintegration. Similarly, Semrud-Clikeman (2010) emphasized the need for family intervention (e.g., provision of information about TBI, such as web-based materials, or a list of community agencies that may be available) at the time of transition from the hospital setting to the home. Another point of transition focused upon was from home to school, with this seen to require the coordination of hospital personnel, family, and school staff (e.g., individual education plan, physical accommodation if necessary, administration of medication, implementation of therapy for emotional and behavioral areas). Planning for life after high school and transition into adulthood was also considered a time for close monitoring and intervention (e.g., integration into higher education, an evaluation of work skills). The authors stressed that challenges may occur at all points of transition, and monitoring and evaluation is needed in order to determine the most appropriate support and intervention.

Dise-Lewis, Lewis, and Reichardt (2009) implemented and evaluated an educational/consultation program for parents and teachers of children with a brain injury. The intervention was known as BrainSTARS (Brain injury: Strategies for Teams and Re-education for Students), an individualized consultation program with a manual specific to pediatric brain injury. A pre-and-post group design was implemented that assessed brain injury-competencies in the adults and also looked at measures of the children's behavior. The intervention comprised three meetings in the school setting. Though the intervention showed improvement in the adults' ability to work with the children, and in the ratings of student performance in targeted neurodevelopmental areas, no change in child behavior was evident.

Community-Based Intervention

Community-based interventions for a pediatric brain injury population are scarce, though recent publications in the adult area, using the Community Approach to Participation (CAP), have shown promising results for community participation (Sloan et al., 2009a,b). This intervention program has shown benefits in the acute and longer term post-injury, in areas including functional independence, community integration, and targeted skills, leading to a reduction in care and support needs.

Chevignard, Toure, Brugel, Poirer, and Laurent-Vannier (2010) described a comprehensive model of care for children following acquired brain injury. Their model discussed the provision of both inpatient and outpatient multidisciplinary rehabilitation, inclusive of on-site specialized schooling, access to long-term follow-up, and the availability of an outreach program. Such an integrated model allows for intervention to occur at different points of transition post-injury with relevant care providers, from childhood to adulthood, when vocational issues are addressed and a referral to adult services can be made.

Sinnakaruppan, Downey, and Morrison (2005) conducted a community-based education program for patients (aged 16–65) and their carers with the aim of improving self-esteem and coping, as well as reducing anxiety and depression in both groups. The intervention addressed problems following brain injury in areas such as memory, executive functioning, and emotion, with training including group discussions, role-playing, and didactic presentations. The intervention length was eight sessions, with assessment at pre-, post-, and three months post-intervention. Though carers showed improvement, this was not statistically significant; however, the patient group did show statistically significant improvement at follow-up, suggesting the need for a larger multi-site study.

A novel approach for intervening in the areas of social and emotional well-being has been presented in a manuscript interested in the implementation of a community-based mentoring program (Fraas & Bellerose, 2010). These authors reported the evaluation of a mentor-adolescent relationship between two survivors of acquired brain injury. The participant was an adolescent survivor of encephalitis, and the mentor a young adult who had sustained a TBI in a motor vehicle accident. The program, established originally for adult survivors of brain injury, showed preliminary results suggesting an enhanced quality of life and psychosocial support for both participants.

Adult Phase: Vocational Intervention

Vocational success, as well as social activity and independent living, are often considered part of community integration or community participation (Sander, Clark, & Pappadis, 2010). As mentioned in the section on community interventions, periods of transition are important points for intervention, especially as the child moves into adulthood and new sets of expectations are experienced (Brenner et al., 2007). With a focus on vocational outcome, the young adult phase may be supported via a range of vocational services, including assistance in the preparation of curriculum vitae and training for higher education and/or job interviews. The individual's needs may also be discussed with potential employers, and site visits may be conducted to determine what environmental modifications may be required (Anderson & Catroppa, 2006).

Asking the question of whether vocational intervention does make a difference in employment outcomes following brain injury, Kendall, Muenchberger, and Gee (2006) conducted a quantitative survey of such research. The sample comprised 3,688 participants who had sustained an injury 16 years and above. Aggregate results showed that return to competitive employment was earlier with vocational intervention and that long-term employment was more achievable for those returning to full-time work. The study also highlighted the issues of definition with regard to employment and optimal time points for measurement of outcome.

Examining the vocational intervention area in more detail, Degeneffe et al. (2008) reported that an initial step would be for vocational counselors to be further educated with regard to TBI, and so be greater advocates for program development, keeping in mind that lifelong challenges would need to be met for this population. It has also been reported that in order to intervene successfully in the vocational area, variables including executive dysfunction, emotional disturbance, impaired daily living, and limited access to rehabilitation services, alongside relevant pre-injury employment status and gender, would have to be addressed (Corrigan, Lineberry, Komaroff, Langlois, et al., 2007; Crepeau & Scherzer, 1993; Walker, Marwitz, Kreutzer, Hart, & Novack, 2006). Similarly, Mateer and Sira (2006) outlined strategies and recommendations for individualized vocational interventions and reported that cognitive rehabilitation strategies that addressed attention, memory, and executive deficits were essential. Improvement in these areas was found to enhance coping skills, as well as cognitive and emotional difficulties, and therefore help the participant meet work demands and expectations.

When examining more detailed approaches to vocational interventions, Fadyl and McPherson (2009), using the principles of a systematic review, identified and evaluated approaches most commonly underpinning such interventions. These authors identified three categories: (i) program-based vocational rehabilitation (focus on jobs skills training); (ii) supported employment; and (iii) case coordination. Though the authors provide a detailed figure to show the features of each model, the key differences between model (ii) and the others was that intervention was delivered entirely while on the job and that the intervention time and extent of intervention was not limited. The main difference between model (iii) and the others was that there was a focus on early intervention and continuity of care, and coordination of vocational rehabilitation with other post-acute rehabilitation services was evident. The authors concluded that, as there was little evidence regarding the efficacy of the models, the proposed framework could be used to evaluate which approach would best suit a particular individual.

An example of a vocational research study with an aim of evaluating the intervention was described by O'Neill, Zuger, Fields, Fraser, and Pruce (2004). These authors implemented a person-centered community-based approach for state rehabilitation counselors to provide vocational rehabilitation (VRehab) services to people with TBI. Participants either were allocated to a traditional approach, where they were referred to various organizations and were monitored by their state VRehab counselor, or were in the treatment group (Program Without Walls—PWW), where they were not referred to outside organizations but received their services from a team of freelance consultants who were recruited, trained, and supervised by the state VRehab counselor overseeing the intervention program. It was found that the PWW intervention was able to place more participants—who worked more hours and for better pay—in comparison to the traditional approach.

Summary

From the preceding literature, it is evident that though interventions may be beneficial in the acute and longer-term phases post-injury, their implementation is fraught with challenges. Though a randomized controlled trial may be considered the gold standard in medical research, this may not always be the best avenue for intervention research. It is often not ethical to place subjects on a waiting list for treatment as is required for such a trial. Furthermore, interventions in general require a substantial time commitment from the participants and their families, different platforms for delivery may be required due to the geographical distribution of families, adaptations are required to suit the age and developmental level of the participants, the best timing of the intervention needs to be determined, the choice of outcome measures to ensure that study effects are captured is an important aspect, and the transfer of skills learned to everyday function is essential. It is clear that the development and implementation of interventions is a challenging area, where an additional difficulty is the lack of evaluation regarding the feasibility and efficacy of the intervention program itself; hence the need for guidelines and classifications to suit different areas of research, in order to establish an evidence base for treatment strategies.

Evaluation of Interventions: A Clinical Perspective

To Treat Cognitive and Behavioral Impairments

Considering the need to evaluate intervention programs, both critical analysis and systematic reviews have been conducted. Gurdin, Huber, and Cochran (2005) conducted a critical analysis of behavioral interventions for children and adolescents with brain injuries in residential and school settings. These authors concluded that the incorporation of a behavioral approach (e.g., antecedents, controls, reinforcement) will more likely result in the achievement of rehabilitation goals; however, it was also highlighted that the next step would be to evaluate the role of behavioral principles. Limond and Leeke (2005) also reviewed published interventions concerning cognitive domains and similarly concluded that though some individual research findings suggest improvements in outcome post-intervention, there was no conclusive evidence for the efficacy of cognitive rehabilitation in the pediatric population, again highlighting the need for more systematically controlled research.

Laatsch and colleagues (2007) undertook a systematic review of cognitive and behavioral rehabilitation treatment studies following acquired brain injury in childhood (0–19 years) between the years 1980 and 2006. Twenty-eight studies met the inclusion criteria and were divided into four treatment domains— (1) comprehensive, (2) attention and memory, (3) speech and language (Sullivan & Riccio, 2010), and (4) behavior. Intervention studies were classified as Class I (high quality) to Class IV (poor quality)—see Table 10.4. Using the standard proposed in the Clinical Practice Guideline Process Manual, which requires evidence from two Class II studies or one Class I study, specific treatment recommendations were made. Of the 28 studies reviewed (1 Class I, 5 Class II, 6 Class III, 16 Class IV) only three evidence-based (1 Classification I, 1 Classification II and III, and 1 Practice Option) recommendations could be made: (i) service providers should provide attention remediation to assist recovery; (ii) comprehensive rehabilitation should involve the family in the intervention process; and (iii) parents or guardians of children seen in emergency would most likely benefit from a TBI information booklet. Issues concerning the variability of the studies available, the diverse intervention techniques and methodologies applied in this field, and the minimal evidence-based recommendations that could be supported were highlighted in this review.

TABLE 10.4 Classification of Intervention Studies

Classification	Criteria
Class I	Prospective randomized control trial (RCT)
	Masked outcome assessment
	Representative population
Class II	Similar to Class I but also include a prospective, matched group cohort
	Without a masked outcome
	Studies with less adequate control procedures
Class III	Well-defined natural history controls or patients serving as their own controls
Class IV	No control group
	Individual case studies
	Clinical case series

Source: Adapted from Laatsch (2007).

Ylvisaker et al. (2007) conducted a systematic review to investigate the effectiveness of behavioral interventions for children and adults with behavior disorders following TBI. Using the classification system above (Laatsch et al., 2007), 64 papers were classified as follows: 1 Class I study; 2 Class II studies; 36 Class III studies; and 25 Class IV studies. Though no practice standards could be made based on Class I or reliable Class II evidence, recommendations made included (1) a Guideline—provision of a behavior intervention (not a specific intervention) for children and adults and (2) an Option—traditional applied behavior analysis (contingency management procedures) and positive behavior interventions and supports may be considered an evidence-based treatment option. This review emphasized the need to embrace a broader mind-set and a different classification system to evaluate research in this area.

A recent systematic review and meta-analysis (Robinson, Kaizar, Catroppa, Godfrey, & Yeates, 2014) examined the effectiveness of cognitive interventions (addressing attention, memory, or executive functions) for children with neurological disorders, acquired brain injuries, and neurodevelopmental disorders. Significant positive treatment effects were found across all domains, but the limited evidence and poor quality of the evidence provided little confidence in the robustness of the meta-analytic results. It was therefore concluded that the results could not be regarded as robust based on the overall poor quality of the evidence and that endorsement of neurocognitive interventions was not warranted without further study.

To Treat Cognitive/Psychosocial Impairments

A systematic review of the literature investigating the effectiveness of psychological interventions aimed at alleviating cognitive and psychosocial difficulties post-pediatric ABI found five cognitive and four psychosocial papers that fit eligibility (Ross, Dorris, & McMillan, 2011). These authors concluded that the literature is limited (cognitive: one high-quality study, three moderate, and one low; psychosocial: one high-quality, two moderate, and one low), but with encouraging results in terms of interventions for reducing attentional and internalizing behavior problems, with further evaluative research required.

To Treat Motor Impairments

When evaluating interventions for the management of motor impairments in a pediatric and adult population post-ABI, Marshall and colleagues (2007) used a classification ranging from "strong evidence" to "consensus opinion." The former required support by two or more randomized controlled trials (RCTs) of fair quality, and the latter an agreement by a group of experts on the appropriate treatment course in the absence of evidence. It was concluded that though a variety of treatment strategies were in use, most were supported by limited (non-randomized controlled trial) evidence.

Issues with the Evaluation of Vocational Intervention

Evaluation of larger-scale interventions, such as vocational interventions, also presents with challenges. Outcomes are difficult to compare due to the types of vocational intervention, the locations of the interventions, the severity of injury of the target group, time post-injury, placement in a new versus a previous job (Hart, Dijkers, White, Braden, et al., 2010), and the need to match an intervention to an individual (Tarazi, Mahone, & Zabel, 2007; Tsaousides & Gordon, 2009), or family (Carey, Wade, & Wolfe, 2008), to optimize success.

Implementation of Research Evidence into Practice

When an intervention has established an evidence base, how is it then implemented into clinical practice? There are a number of factors that may prove to be a barrier to the implementation of the program, and these may include a mismatch with clinician practices, the family's lack of understanding of brain injury and the benefits of the program, lack of support of the health agency, and inadequate staff numbers. Alternatively, there are factors that may facilitate the implementation of a program into clinical care, such as gaining information about the service where the intervention is to be implemented (characteristics of the adopters), determining whether there is a match between the culture and needs of the service and the intervention, and ensuring the intensity and duration of training is practical and feasible (e.g., will this lead to an efficient service and a satisfied client?). The implementation process is essential for the availability of evidence-based programs to those in need (Fixsen, Naoom, Blase, Friedman, & Wallace, 2005).

Considerations

Despite hurdles in the development, methodology, implementation, and evaluation of research in the rehabilitation area, and with literature on interventions and efficacy minimal in both child and adult areas (Gordon, Zafonte, Cicerone, Cantor, et al., 2006), current evidence does suggest that intervention post-TBI is beneficial (Tsaousides & Gordon, 2009), motivating researchers to continue strengthening and expanding this area. However, there remains the need for well-developed studies to examine the efficacy of these interventions, with more specific studies often lacking generalizability, and more holistic studies presenting with difficulty in isolating the effective components and standardizing the intervention (Slomine & Locascio, 2009).

As mentioned previously, traditionally, the most appropriate design for treatment evaluation (taking into account factors such as ongoing development in the child and spontaneous recovery) is the randomized controlled trial (RCT). Though there are some advantages with RCTs, when working with a TBI population, ethical considerations (e.g., delaying treatment if one is assigned to a wait-list control group) often preclude the use of a RCT design, and some research questions in brain injury are better suited to a social model of disability (Malec, 2009) than a medical model. Including multiple research designs in child TBI is crucial in providing important information regarding the efficacy of the implemented intervention (Slifer & Amari, 2009). Studies that allow for clinically relevant research—in particular, carefully designed single case studies, where the methodology can be rated and statistical techniques can be applied to measure efficacy (Perdices & Tate, 2009)—need to be implemented to further knowledge in the field.

Conclusions

There are many hurdles in developing and evaluating the effects of an intervention. These may include accounting for spontaneous recovery, the use of limited and inappropriate outcome measures, the different operationalization of measures across studies, differing study methodologies, small sample sizes, the decision regarding when intervention is most efficacious and safe, and how long to continue treatment. Interventions may target an area of cognitive impairment or be implemented at the broader level of participation (Whyte, 2009), and, often, due to such complexity, multiple methods and models incorporating diverse methodologies (e.g., biopsychosocial model) may need to be integrated to ensure the best outcome for the individual (Gracey, Evans, & Malley, 2009). Due to these hurdles, the literature presents intervention programs that often lack a strong evidence base, highlighting the need for further quality research. Further challenges are faced at the implementation stage, where it is essential that barriers are reduced and facilitators strengthened, in order for evidence-based intervention programs to be used in clinical care, bridging a gap that is present in the health-care system for a pediatric population following brain injury. Efficacious interventions across the life span will lead to reduced cost to the larger society and, most importantly, to improved quality of life for the individuals with TBI and their families. There is still much work to be done in this field.

REFERENCES

Aaen, G. S., Holshouser, B. A., Sheridan, C., Colbert, C., McKenney, M., Kido, D., & Ashwal, S. (2010). Magnetic resonance spectroscopy predicts outcomes for children with nonaccidental trauma. *Pediatrics, 125*(2), 295–303.

Aaro Jonsson, C., Smedler, A. C., Leis Ljungmark, M., & Emanuelson, I. (2009). Long-term cognitive outcome after neurosurgically treated childhood traumatic brain injury. *Brain Injury, 23*(13–14), 1008–1016.

Access Economics. (2009). *The economic cost of spinal cord injury and traumatic brain injury in Australia.* Report by Access Economics Pty Limited for the Victorian Neurotrauma Initiative.

Achenbach, T. M., & Edelbrock, C. (1991). Child behavior checklist. Burlington (Vt) 7.61: University of Vermont, Research Center for Children, Youth, & Families.

Achenbach, T. M., Thomas, M., & Rescorla, L. A. (2001). *Manual for the ASEBA School-Age Forms & Profiles.* Burlington, VT: University of Vermont, Research Center for Children, Youth, & Families.

Adams, J., Frumiento, C., Shatney-Leach, L., & Vane, D. (2001). Mandatory admission after isolated mild closed head injury in children: Is it necessary? *Journal of Pediatric Surgery, 36,* 119–121.

Adamson, C., Yuan, W., Babcock, L., Leach, J. L., Seal, M. L., Holland, S. K., & Wade, S. L. (2013). Diffusion tensor imaging detects white matter abnormalities and associated cognitive deficits in chronic adolescent TBI. *Brain Injury, 27*(4), 454–463.

Adelson, P. D. (2009). Hypothermia following pediatric traumatic brain injury. *Journal of Neurotrauma, 26,* 429–436.

Adelson, P. D. (2010). Clinical trials for pediatric TBI. In V. A. Anderson & K. O. Yeates (Eds.), *New directions in pediatric traumatic brain injury: Multidisciplinary and translational perspectives* (pp. 54–67). New York, NY: Oxford University Press.

Adelson, P. D., Bratton, S. L., Carney, N. A., Chesnut, R. M., du Coudray, H. E., Goldstein, B. . . . Wright, D. W. (2003). *Guidelines for the acute medical management of severe traumatic brain injury in infants, children, and adolescents.* Chapter 1: Introduction. *Pediatric Critical Care Medicine, 4* (suppl. 3), S2–S4.

Adelson, D., & Kochanek, P. (1998). Head injury in children. *Journal of Child Neurology, 13*, 2–15.

Adelson, P. D., Nemoto, E., Colak, A., & Painter, M. (1998). The use of near infrared spectroscopy (NIRS) in children after traumatic brain injury: A preliminary report. *Acta Neurochir Suppl, 71*, 250–254.

Adelson, P., Ragheb, J., Muizelaar, J., Kaney, P., Brockmeyer, D., Beers, S. R., . . . Levin, H. (2005). Phase II clinical trial of moderate hypothermia after severe traumatic brain injury in children. *Neurosurgery, 56*(4), 740–754.

Agrawal, A., Timothy, J., Pandit, L., & Manju, M. (2006). Post-traumatic epilepsy: An overview. *Clinical Neurology and Neurosurgery, 108*(5), 433–439.

Alves, W. (1992). Natural history of post-concussive signs and symptoms. *Physical Medicine and Rehabilitation: State of the Arts Reviews, 6*, 21–32.

Alzaga, A. G., Cerdan, M., & Varon, J. (2007). Therapeutic hypothermia. *Resuscitation, 70*, 369–380.

Amacher, A. L. (1988). *Paediatric head injuries: A handbook.* St. Louis, MO: Warren H. Green, Inc.

American Speech-Language-Hearing Association. (2004). *Preferred Practice Patterns for the Profession of Speech-Language Pathology.* Retrieved from www.asha.org/policy

An, M., & Palisano, R. J. (2013). Family-professional collaboration in pediatric rehabilitation: A practice model. *Disability and Rehabilitation, Early Online,* 1–7.

Anderson, P. (2002). Assessment and development of executive function (EF) during childhood. *Child Neuropsychology, 8*, 71–82.

Anderson, V. (2003). Outcome and management of traumatic brain injury in childhood. In B. Wilson (Ed.), *Neuropsychological rehabilitation: Theory and practice* (pp. 217–252). Lisse, The Netherlands: Swets & Zeitlinger.

Anderson, V., Anderson, P., Northam, E., Jacobs, R., & Catroppa, C. (2001). Development of executive functions through late childhood and adolescence in an Australian sample. *Developmental Neuropsychology, 20*, 385–406.

Anderson, V., Brown, S., & Newitt, H. (2010). What contributes to quality of life in adult survivors of childhood traumatic brain injury? *Journal of Neurotrauma, 27*(5), 863–870.

Anderson, V., Brown, S., Newitt, H., & Hoile, H. (2009). Educational, vocational, psychosocial and quality of life outcomes for adult survivors of childhood traumatic brain injury. *Journal of Head Trauma Rehabilitation, 24*(5), 303–312.

Anderson, V., Brown, S., Newitt, H., & Hoile, H. (2011). Long-term outcome from childhood traumatic brain injury: Intellectual ability, personality, and quality of life. *Neuropsychology, 25*(2), 176–184.

Anderson, V., & Catroppa, C. (2005). Recovery of executive skills following paediatric traumatic brain injury (TBI): A 2 year follow-up. *Brain Injury, 19*(6), 459–470.

Anderson, V., & Catroppa, C. (2006). Advances in postacute rehabilitation after childhood acquired brain injury: A focus on cognitive, behavioral, and social domains. *American Journal of Physical Medicine and Rehabilitation, 85*(9), 767–787.

Anderson, V., Catroppa, C., Dudgeon, P., Morse, S., Haritou, F., & Rosenfeld, J. (2006). Understanding predictors of functional recovery and outcome 30 months following early childhood head injury. *Neuropsychology, 20*(1), 42–57.

Anderson, V., Catroppa, C., Haritou, F., Morse, S., & Rosenfeld, J. (2005). Identifying factors contributing to child and family outcome at 30 months following traumatic brain injury in children. *Journal of Neurology, Neurosurgery and Psychiatry, 76*, 401–408.

Anderson, V., Morse, S., Catroppa, C., Haritou, F., & Rosenfeld, J. (2004). Thirty month outcome from early childhood head injury: A prospective analysis of neurobehavioural recovery. *Brain, 127*, 2608–2620.

Anderson, V., Catroppa, C., Morse, S., Haritou, F., & Rosenfeld, J. (2000). Recovery of intellectual ability following traumatic brain injury in childhood: Impact of injury severity and age at injury. *Pediatric Neurosurgery, 32*(6), 282–290.

Anderson, V., Catroppa, C., Morse, S., Haritou, F., & Rosenfeld, J. (2001). Outcome from mild head injury in young children: A prospective study. *Journal of Clinical and Experimental Neuropsychology, 23*(6), 705–717.

Anderson, V, Catroppa, C., Morse, S., Haritou, F., & Rosenfeld, J. (2005). Attentional and processing skills following traumatic brain injury in early childhood. *Brain Injury, 19*(9), 699–710.

Anderson, V., Catroppa, C., Morse, S., Haritou, F., & Rosenfeld, J. (2005a). Functional plasticity or vulnerability after early brain injury? *Pediatrics, 116*(6), 1374–1382.

Anderson, V., Catroppa, C., Morse, S., Haritou, F., & Rosenfeld, J. (2005b). Attentional and processing skills following traumatic brain injury in early childhood. *Brain Injury, 19*(9), 699–710.

Anderson, V., Catroppa, C., Morse, S., Haritou, F., & Rosenfeld, J. V. (2010). Intellectual outcome from preschool traumatic brain injury: A 5-year prospective, longitudinal study. *Pediatrics, 124*, e1064–1071.

Anderson, V., Godfrey, C., Rosenfeld, J. V., & Catroppa, C. (2011). Intellectual ability 10 years after traumatic brain injury in infancy and childhood: What predicts outcome? *Journal of Neurotrauma, 29*(1), 143–153.

Anderson, V., & Moore, C. (1995). Age at injury as a predictor of outcome following pediatric head injury: A longitudinal perspective. *Child Neuropsychology, 1*(3), 187–202.

Anderson, V. A., Morse, S. A., Catroppa, C., Haritou, F., & Rosenfeld, J. V. (2004). Thirty month outcome from early childhood head injury: A prospective analysis of neurobehavioural recovery. *Brain, 127*, 2608–2620.

Anderson, V. A., Morse, S., Klug, G., Catroppa, C., Haritou, F., Rosenfeld, J., & Pentland, L. (1997). Predicting recovery from head injury in young children: A prospective analysis. *Journal of the International Neuropsychological Society, 3*, 568–580.

Anderson, V., Northam, E., Hendy, J., & Wrennall, J. (2001). *Developmental neuropsychology: A clinical approach.* New York, NY: Psychology Press.

Anderson, V., & Pentland, L. (1998). Residual attention deficits following childhood head injury: Implications for ongoing development. *Neuropsychological Rehabilitation, 8*(3), 283–300.

Anderson, V., Spencer-Smith, M., Leventer, R., Coleman, L., Anderson, P., Williams, J., . . . Jacobs, R. (2009). Childhood brain insult: Can age at insult help us predict outcome? *Brain, 132*(1), 45–56.

Anderson, V., & Yeates, K. O. (Eds.). (2010). *Pediatric traumatic brain injury: New frontiers in clinical and translational research.* Cambridge, UK: Cambridge University Press.

Andersson, E., Sejdhage, R., & Wage, V. (2012). Mild traumatic brain injuries in children between 0–16 years of age: A survey of activities and places when an accident occurs. *Developmental Neurorehabilitation, 15*(1), 26–30.

Andrews, T. K., Rose, F. D., & Johnson, D. A. (1998). Social and behavioural effects of traumatic brain injury in children. *Brain Injury, 12*(2), 133–138.

Andriessen, T., Jacobs, B., & Vos, E. (2010). Clinical characteristics and pathophysiological mechanisms of focal and diffuse traumatic brain injury. *J Cell Mol Med, 14*(10), 2381–2392.

Annegers, J. F. (1983). The epidemiology of head trauma in children. In K. Shapiro (Ed.), *Pediatric head trauma* (pp. 1–10). Mount Kisco, NY: Futura.

Anon. (2015). Sport Concussion Assessment Tool (3rd ed.).*Brit J Sports Med*. Retrieved from http://bjsm.bmj.com/content/47/5/259.full.pdf

Anson, K., & Ponsford, J. (2006). Coping and emotional adjustment following traumatic brain injury. *Journal of Head Trauma Rehabilitation, 21*(3), 248–259.

Antonini, T. N., Raj, S. P., Oberjohn, K. S., & Wade, S. L. (2012). An online positive parent-ing skills program for paediatric traumatic brain injury: Feasibility and parental satisfac-tion. *Journal of Telemedicine and Telecare, 18*, 333–338.

Arango, J. I., Deibert, C. P., Brown, D., Bell, M., Dvorchik, I., & Adelson, P. D. (2012). Post-traumatic seizures in children with severe traumatic brain injury. *Child's Nerv Syst, 28*(11), 1925–1929.

Arco, L., & Bishop, J. (2009). Single participant studies in positive behavior support for parents of individuals with brain injuries. *Brain Impairment, 10*(3), 307–319.

Aronowski, J., & Zhao, X. (2011). Molecular pathophysiology of cerebral hemorrhage: Secondary brain injury. *Stroke, 42*, 1781–1786.

Asarnow, R. F., Satz, P., Light, R., Lewis, R., & Neumann, E. (1991). Behavior problems and adaptive functioning in children with mild and severe closed head injury. *Journal of Pediatric Psychology, 16*, 543–555.

Asarnow, R. F., Satz, P., Light, R., Zaucha, K., Lewis, R., & McCleary, C. (1995). The UCLA study of mild closed head injuries in children and adolescents. In S. H. Broman & M. E. Michel (Eds.), *Traumatic head injury in children* (pp. 117–146). New York, NY: Oxford University Press.

Ashwal, S. (2004). Pediatric vegetative state: Epidemiological and clinical issues. *NeuroReha-bilitation, 19*(4), 349–360.

Ashwal, S., Babikian, T., Gardner-Nichols, J., Freier, M. C., Tong, K. A., & Holshouser, B. A. (2006). Susceptibility-weighted imaging and proton magnetic resonance spectroscopy in assessment of outcome after pediatric traumatic brain injury. *Arch Phys Med Rehabil, 87*(12 Suppl), 50–58.

Ashwal, S., Holshouser, B. A., & Tong, K. A. (2006). Use of advanced neuroimaging tech-niques in the evaluation of pediatric traumatic brain injury. *Dev Neurosci, 28*(4–5), 309–326.

Ashwal, S., Holshouser, B., Tong, K., Serna, T., Osterdock, R., Gross, M., & Kido, D. (2004). Proton MR spectroscopy detected glutamate/glutamine is increased in children with traumatic brain injury. *Journal of Neurotrauma, 21*(11), 1539–1552.

Ashwal, S., Tong, K. A., Bartnik-Olson, B., & Holshouser, B. A. (2012). Neuroimaging. In M. W. Kirkwood & K. O. Yeates (Eds.), *Mild traumatic brain injury in children and adolescents: From basic science to clinical management* (pp. 162–195). New York, NY: Guilford Press.

Asikainen, I., Nybo, T., Muller, K., Sarna, S., & Kaste, M. (1999). Speed performance and long-term functional and vocational outcome in a group of young patients with moder-ate or severe traumatic brain injury. *European Journal of Neurology, 6*(2), 179–185.

Aubry, M., Cantu, R., Dvorak, J., Graf-Baumann, T., Johnston, K., Kelly, J., . . . Schamasch, P. (2002). Summary and agreement statement on the first international conferecne on concussion in sport, Vienna 2001. *British Journal of Sports Medicine, 36*, 6–17.

Ayr, L. K., Yeates, K. O., Taylor, H. G., & Browne, M. (2009). Dimensions of postconcussive symptoms in children with mild traumatic brain injuries. *J Int Neuropsychol Soc, 15*(1), 19–30.

Babikian, T., & Asarnow, R. (2009). Neurocognitive outcomes and recovery after pediatric TBI: Meta-analytic review of the literature. *Neuropsychology, 23*(3), 283–296.

Babikian, T., Freier, C. M., Asher, S., Riggs, M. T., Burley, T., & Holshouser, B. A. (2006). MR spectroscopy: Predicting long-term neuropsychological outcome following pedia-tric TBI. *Journal of Magnetic Resonance Imaging, 24*, 801–811.

Babikian, T., Freier, M. C., Tong, K. A., Nickerson, J. P., Wall, C. J., Holshouser, B. A., . . . Ashwal S. (2005). Susceptibility weighted imaging: Neuropsychologic outcome and pediatric head injury. *Pediatric Neurology, 33*(3), 184–194.

Babikian, T., Marion, S. D., Copeland, S., Alger, J. R., O'Neill, J., Cazalis, F., . . . Asarnow, R. F. (2010). Metabolic levels in the corpus callosum and their structural and behavioral correlates after moderate to severe pediatric TBI. *Journal of Neurotrauma, 27*(3), 473–481.

Babikian, T., McArthur, D., & Asarnow, R. F. (2012). Predictors of 1-month and 1-year neurocognitive functioning from the UCLA longitudinal mild, uncomplicated, pediatric traumatic brain injury study. *Journal of the International Neuropsychological Society, 18*, 1–10.

Babikian, T., Satz, P., Zaucha, K., Light, R., Lewic, R. S., & Asarnow, R. F. (2011). The UCLA longitudinal study of neurocognitive outcomes following mild pediatric traumatic brain injury. *Journal of the International Neuropsychological Society, 17*, 886–895.

Baddeley, A. (1990). *Human memory: Theory and practice.* Oxford: Oxford University Press.

Baker, F. (2001). The effects of live, taped, and no music on people experiencing posttraumatic amnesia. *Journal of Music Therapy, 38*, 170–192.

Bakker, K., & Waugh, M. C. (2000). Stimulant use in paediatric acquired brain injury: Evaluation of a protocol. *Brain Impairment, 1*, 29–36

Barca, L., Cappelli, F. R., Amicuzi, I., Apicella, M. G., Castelli, E., & Stortini, M. (2009). Modality-specific naming impairment after traumatic brain injury (TBI). *Brain Injury, 23*(11), 920–929.

Barkhoudarian, G., Hovda, D., & Giza, C. (2011). The molecular pathophysiology of concussive brain injury. *Clinical Sports Medicine, 30*, 33–48.

Barlow, K., Crawford, S., Stevenson, A., Sandhu, S. S., Belanger, F., & Dewey, D. (2010). Epidemiology of postconcussional syndrome in pediatric mild traumatic brain injury. *Pediatrics, 126*(2), 374–381.

Barnes, M. A., Dennis, M., & Wilkinson, M. (1999). Reading after closed head injury in childhood. Effects on accuracy, fluency, and comprehension. *Developmental Neuropsychology, 15*(1), 1–24.

Barnes, P. D. (2011). Imaging of nonaccidental injury and the mimics: Issues and controversies in the era of evidence-based medicine. *Radiologic Clinics of North America, 49*(1), 205–229.

Baron, I. S. (2004). *Neuropsychological evaluation of the child.* Oxford: Oxford University Press.

Bayir, H., Adelson, P. D., Wisniewski, S. R., Shore, P., Lai, Y., Brown, D., . . . Kochanek, P. M. (2009). Therapeutic hypothermia preserves antioxidant defenses after severe traumatic brain injury in infants and children. *Critical Care and Medicine, 37*, 2, 689–695.

Bayley, N. (2005). *The Bayley Scales of Infant Development* (3rd ed.). San Antonio, TX: Psychological Corporation.

Beardmore, S., Tate, R., & Liddle, B. (1999). Does information and feedback improve children's knowledge and awareness of deficits after traumatic brain injury? *Neuropsychological Rehabilitation, 9*, 45–62.

Beauchamp, M. H., & Anderson, V. (2010). SOCIAL: An integrative framework for the development of social skills. *Psychological Bulletin, 136*(1), 39–64.

Beauchamp, M. H., Anderson, V. A., Catroppa, C., Maller, J. J., Godfrey, C., Rosenfeld, J. V., & Kean, M. (2009). Implications of reduced callosal area for social skills after severe traumatic brain injury in children. *Journal of Neurotrauma, 26*(10), 1645–1654.

Beauchamp, M. H., Anderson, V., Catroppa, C., Maller, J. J., Godfrey, C., Rosenfeld, J. V., . . . Anderson, V. (2011). Hippocampus, amygdala and global brain changes 10 years after childhood traumatic brain injury. *International Journal of Developmental Neuroscience, 29*, 137–143.

Beauchamp, M. H., Beare, R., Ditchfield, M., Coleman, L., Babl, F. E., Kean, M., . . . Anderson, V. (2013). Susceptibility weighted imaging and its relationship to outcome after pediatric traumatic brain injury. *Cortex, 49*(2), 591–598.

Beauchamp, M. H., Catroppa, C., Godfrey, C., Morse, S., Rosenfeld. J. V., & Anderson, V. A. (2011). Selective executive deficits ten years after severe childhood traumatic brain injury. *Developmental Neuropsychology, 36*(5), 578–595.

Beauchamp, M. H., Ditchfield, M., Babl, F. E., Kean, M., Catroppa, C., Yeates, K. O., & Anderson, V. (2011). Detecting traumatic brain lesions in children: CT versus MRI versus Susceptibility Weighted Imaging (SWI). *Journal of Neurotrauma, 28*(6), 915–927.

Beauchamp, M. H., Ditchfield, M., Catroppa, C., Kean, M., Godfrey, C., Rosenfeld, J. V., & Anderson, V. (2011). Focal thinning of the posterior corpus callosum: Normal variant or post-traumatic? *Brain Injury, 25*(10), 950–957.

Beauchamp, M.H., Ditchfield, M., Maller, J.J. Catroppa, C., Godfrey, C., Rosenfeld, J.V., Kean, M.J., & Anderson, V. (2011). Hippocampus, amygdala and global brain changes 10 years after childhood traumatic brain injury. *International Journal of Developmental Neuroscience, 29*, 137–143.

Beauchamp, M. H., Dooley, J. J., & Anderson, V. (2010). Adult outcomes of childhood traumatic brain injury. In J. Donders & S. Hunter (Eds.), *Principles and practice of lifespan developmental neuropsychology* (pp. 315–328). Cambridge, UK: Cambridge University Press.

Beauchamp, M. H., Dooley, J. J., & Anderson, V. (2013). A preliminary investigation of moral reasoning and empathy after traumatic brain injury in adolescents. *Brain Injury, 27*(7–8), 896–902.

Beaudin, M., Saint-Vil, D., Ouimet, A., Mercier, C., & Crevier, L. (2007). Clinical algorithm and resource use in the management of children with minor head trauma. *Journal of Pediatric Surgery, 42*(5), 849–852.

Bedell, G. M. (2008). Functional outcomes of school-age children with acquired injuries at discharge from inpatient rehabilitation. *Brain Injury, 22*(4), 313–324.

Bedell, G. (2009). Further validation of the Child and Adolescent Scale of Participation (CASP). *Developmental Neurorehabilitation, 12*(5), 342–351.

Bedell, G. M., Cohn, E. S., & Dumas, H. M. (2005). Exploring parents' use of strategies to promote social participation of school-age children with acquired brain injuries. *The American Journal of Occupational Therapy, 59*(3), 273–284.

Beers, S. R. (1992). Cognitive effect of mild head injury in children and adolescents. *Neuropsychology Review, 3*, 281–320.

Beers, S. R., Skold, A., Dixon, C. E., & Adelson, P. D. (2005). Neurobehavioral effects of amantadine after pediatric traumatic brain injury. *Journal of Head Trauma Rehabilitation, 20*(5), 450–463.

Begali, V. (1992). *Head injury in children and adolescents* (2nd ed.). Brandon, VT: Clinical Psychology Publishing Company Inc.

Belanger, H. G., Vanderploeg, R. D., Curtiss, G., & Warden, D. L. (2007). Recent neuroimaging techniques in mild traumatic brain injury. *J Neuropsychiatry Clin Neurosci, 19*(1), 5–20.

Bell, M. J., & Kochanek, P. M. (2008). Traumatic brain injury in children: Recent advances in management. *Indian Journal of Pediatrics, 75*, 1159–1165.

Bell, M. J., & Kochanek, P. M. (2013). Pediatric traumatic brain injury in 2012: The year with new guidelines and common data elements. *Critical Care Clinics, 29*, 223–238.

Benn, K. M., & McColl, M. A. (2004). Parental coping following childhood acquired brain injury. *Brain Injury, 18*(3), 239–255.

Benson, R. R., Meda, S. A., Vasudevan, S., Kou, Z., Govindarajan, K. A., Hanks, R. A., . . . Haacke, E. M. (2007). Global white matter analysis of diffusion tensor images is predictive of injury severity in traumatic brain injury. *Journal of Neurotrauma, 24*(3), 446–459.

Berger, R. P. (2006). The use of serum biomarkers to predict outcome after traumatic brain injury in adults and children. *J Head Trauma Rehabil, 21*(4), 315–333.

Berger, R. P., Beers, S. R., Richichi, R., Wiesman, D., & Adelson, P. D. (2007). Serum biomarker concentrations and outcome after pediatric traumatic brain injury. *Journal of Neurotrauma, 24*(12), 1793–1801.

Berger, R. P., Dulani, T., Adelson, P. D., Leventhal, J. M., Richichi, R., & Kochanek, P. M. (2006). Identification of inflicted traumatic brain injury in well-appearing infants using serum and cerebrospinal markers: A possible screening tool. *Pediatrics, 117*(2), 325–332.

Berger, R. P., Kochanek, P. M., & Pierce, M. C. (2004). Biochemical markers of brain injury: Could they be used as diagnostic adjuncts in cases of inflicted traumatic brain injury? *Child Abuse Negl, 28*(7), 739–754.

Berger, R. P., Ta'asan, S., Rand, A., Lokshin, A., & Kochanek, P. (2009). Multiplex assessment of serum biomarker concentrations in well-appearing children with inflicted traumatic brain injury. *Pediatric Research, 65*(1), 97–102.

Berger, R. P., & Zuckerbraun, N. (2012). Biochemical markers. In M. W. Kirkwood & K. O. Yeates (Eds.), *Mild traumatic brain injury in children and adolescents: From basic science to clinical management* (pp. 145–161). New York, NY: Guilford Press.

Berger-Gross, P., & Shackelford, M. (1985). Closed-head injury in children: Neuropsychological and scholastic outcomes. *Perceptual and Motor Skills, 61*, 254.

Berney, J., Favier, J., & Froidevaux, A. (1994). Pediatric head trauma: Influence of age and sex. I. Epidemiology. *Child's Nervous System, 10*, 509–516.

Betts, J., McKay, J., Maruff, P., & Anderson, V. (2006). The development of sustained attention in children: The effect of age and task load. *Child Neuropsychology, 12*(3), 205–221.

Bhambhani, Y., Maikala, R., Farag, M., & Rowland, G. (2006). Reliability of near-infrared spectroscopy measures of cerebral oxygenation and blood volume during handgrip exercise in nondisabled and traumatic brain-injured subjects. *Journal of Rehabilitation Research and Development, 43*(7), 845–856.

Biddle, K. R., McCabe, A., & Bliss, L. S. (1996). Narrative skills following traumatic brain injury in children and adults. *Journal of Communication Disorders, 29*, 447–469.

Bigler, E. D. (1999). Neuroimaging in pediatric traumatic head injury: Diagnostic considerations and relationships to neurobehavioral outcome. *J Head Trauma Rehabil, 14*(4), 406–423.

Bigler, E. D. (2007). Anterior and middle cranial fossa in traumatic brain injury: Relevant neuroanatomy and neuropathology in the study of neuropsychological outcome. *Neuropsychology, 21*, 515–31.

Bigler, E. D., Abildskov, T. J., Petrie, J., Farrer, T. J., Dennis, M., Simic, N., . . . Yeates, K. O. (2013). Heterogeneity of brain lesions in pediatric traumatic brain injury. *Neuropsychology, 27*(4), 438–451.

Bigler, E. D., Abildskov, T. J., Wilde, E. A., McCauley, S. R., Li, X., Merkley, T. L. . . . Levin, H. S. (2010). Diffuse damage in pediatric traumatic brain injury: A comparison of automated versus operator-controlled quantification methods. *Neuroimage, 50*(3), 1017–1026.

Bigler, E. D., & Maxwell, W. L. (2011). Neuroimaging and neuropathology of TBI. *NeuroRehabilitation, 28*, 63–74.

Bijur, P., Goulding, J., Haslum, M., & Kurzon, M. (1988). Behavioral predictors of injury in school-aged children. *American Journal of Diseases in Childhood, 142*, 1307–1312.

Bin, S. S., Schutzman, S. A., & Greenes, D. S. (2010). Validation of a clinical score to predict skull fracture in head-injured infants. *Pediatric Emergency Care, 26*(9), 633–639.

Biswas, A. K., Bruce, D. A., Sklar, F. H., Bokovoy, J. L., & Sommerauer, J. F. (2002). Treatment of acute traumatic brain injury in children with moderate hypothermia improves intracranial hypertension. *Critical Care and Medicine, 30,* 2742–2751.

Blackman, J. A., Worley, G., & Strittmatter, W. J. (2005). Apolipoprotein E and brain injury: Implications for children. *Developmental Medicine & Child Neurology, 47,* 64–70.

Blakemore, S. (2010). The developing social brain: Implications for education. *Neuron, 65*(6), 744–747.

Bloom, D. R., Levin, H. S., Ewing-Cobbs, L., Saunders, A. E., Song, J., & Fletcher, J. M. (2001). Lifetime and novel psychiatric disorders after pediatric traumatic brain injury. *Journal of the American Academy of Child and Adolescent Psychiatry, 40*(5), 572–579.

Bohnert, A. M., Parker, J. G., & Warschausky, S. A. (1997). Friendship and social adjustment following a traumatic brain injury: An exploratory investigation. *Developmental Neuropsychology, 13,* 477–486.

Boll, T. J. (1983). Minor head injury in children: Out of sight but not out of mind. *Journal of Clinical Child and Adolescent Psychology, 12*(1), 74–80.

Bower, J. (2010). Music therapy for a 10-year old child experiencing agitation during post-traumatic amnesia: An intrinsic mixed methods case study. Master's Dissertation (Master of Music), University of Melbourne, Melbourne, Victoria, Australia.

Bowman, S. M., Bird, T. M., Aitken, M. E., & Tilford, J. M. (2008). Trends in hospitalizations associated with pediatric traumatic brain injuries. *Pediatrics, 122,* 988–993.

Braga, L. W., Da Paz, A. C. Jr., & Ylvisaker, M. (2005). Direct clinician-delivered versus indirect family-supported rehabilitation of children with traumatic brain injury: A randomized controlled trial. *Brain Injury, 19*(10), 819–831.

Brenner, D. J. (2010). Should we be concerned about the rapid increase in CT usage? *Reviews on Environmental Health, 25*(1), 63–68.

Brenner, D., Elliston, C., Hall, E., & Berdon, W. (2001). Estimated risks of radiation-induced fatal cancer from pediatric CT. *AJR Am J Roentgenol, 176*(2), 289–296.

Brenner, L. A., Dise-Lewis, J. E., Bartles, S. K., O'Brien, S. E., Godleski, M., & Selinger, M. (2007). The long-term impact and rehabilitation of pediatric traumatic brain injury: A 50-year follow-up case study. *Journal of Head Trauma Rehabilitation, 22*(1), 56–64.

Brenner, T., Freier, M. C., Holshouser, B. A., Burley, T., & Ashwal, S. (2003). Predicting neuropsychologic outcome after traumatic brain injury in children. *Pediatr Neurol, 28*(2), 104–114.

Breslau, N. (1990). Does brain dysfunction increase children's vulnerability to environmental stress? *Archives of General Psychiatry, 47,* 15–20.

Brett, A. W., & Laatsch, L. (1998). Cognitive rehabilitation therapy of brain-injured students in a public high school setting. *Pediatric Rehabilitation, 2,* 27–31.

Brewer, K., Pollock, N., & Virginia Wright, F. (2013). Addressing the challenges of collaborative goal setting with children and their families. *Physical and Occupational Therapy in Pediatrics, Early Online,* 1–15.

Broglio, S. P., & Puetz, T. W. (2008). The effect of sports concussion on neurocognitive function, self-report symptoms and postural control—A meta-analysis. *Sports Medicine, 38,* 53–67.

Brooks, D. N., Aughton, M. E., Bond, M. R., Jones, P., & Rizvi, S. (1980). Cognitive sequelae in relationship to early indices of severity of brain damage after severe blunt head injury. *Journal of Neurology, Neurosurgery and Psychiatry, 43*(6), 529–534.

Brown, G., Chadwick, O., Shaffer, D., Rutter, M., & Traub, M. (1981). A prospective study of children with head injuries: III. Psychiatric sequelae. *Psychological Medicine, 11*(1), 63–78.

Browne, G. J., & Lam, L. T. (2008). Concussive head injury in children and adolescents related to sports and other leisure physical activities. *British Journal of Sports Medicine, 40*, 163–168.

Browning, J. G., Reed, M. J., Wilkinson, A. G., & Beattie, T. (2005). Imaging infants with head injury: Effect of a change in policy. *Emerg Med J, 22*(1), 33–36.

Bruce, D. A. (1995). Pathophysiological responses of the child's brain. In S. H. Broman & M. E. Michel (Eds.), *Traumatic head injury in children* (pp. 40–51). New York, NY: Oxford University Press.

Bruce, J., Echemendia, R., Meeuwisse, W., Comper, P., & Sisco, A. (2014). 1 year test-retest reliability of ImPACT in professional ice hockey players. *Clin Neuropsychol, 28*(1), 14–25.

Bruneau-Bhérer, R., Achim, A. M., & Jackson, P. L. (2012). Measuring the different components of social cognition in children and adolescents. In V. Anderson & M. H. Beauchamp (Eds.), *Developmental social neuroscience and childhood brain insult: Theory and practice* (pp. 138–160). New York, NY: Guilford Press.

Bryck, R. L., & Fisher, P. A. (2012). Training the brain. Practical applications of neural plasticity from the intersection of cognitive neuroscience, developmental psychology and prevention science. *American Psychologist, 67*(2), 87–100.

Burke, W. H., Wesolowski, M. D., & Guth, M. L. (1988). Comprehensive head injury rehabilitation: An outcome evaluation. *Brain Injury, 2*(4), 313–322.

Buttram, S.D.W., Wisniewski, S. R., Jackson, E. K., Adelson, P. D., Feldman, K., Bayir, H. . . . Kochanek, P. M. (2007). Multiplex assessment of cytokine and chemokine levels in cerebrospinal fluid following severe pediatric traumatic brain injury: Effects of moderate hypothermia. *Journal of Neurotrauma, 24*, 43–53.

Byard, K., Fine, H., & Reed, J. (2011). Taking a developmental and systematic perspective on neuropsychological rehabilitation with children with brain injury and their families. *Clinical Child Psychology and Psychiatry, 16*(2), 165–184.

Byars, A. W., Holland, S. K., Strawsburg, R. H., Bommer, W., Dunn, R. S., Schmithorst, V. J., & Plante, E. (2002). Practical aspects of conducting large-scale functional magnetic resonance imaging studies in children. *Journal of Child Neurology, 17*(12), 885–890.

Caeyenberghs, K., Leemans, A., Geurts, M., Taymans, T., Vander Linden, C., Smits-Engelsman, B. C., . . . Swinnen, S. P. (2010). Brain-behavior relationships in young traumatic brain injury patients: Fractional anisotropy measures are highly correlated with dynamic visuomotor tracking performance. *Neuropsychologia, 48*(5), 1472–1482.

Caeyenberghs, K., Wenderoth, N., Smits-Engelsman, B. C., Sunaert, S., & Swinnen, S. P. (2009). Neural correlates of motor dysfunction in children with traumatic brain injury: Exploration of compensatory recruitment patterns. *Brain, 132*(Pt 3), 684–694.

Campbell, T. F., & Dollaghan, C. A. (1990). Expressive language recovery in severely brain injured children and adolescents. *Journal of Speech and Hearing Disorders, 55*, 567–586.

Capruso, D. X., & Levin, H. S. (1992). Cognitive impairment following closed head injury. *Neurologic Clinics, 10*(4), 879–893.

Carey, J. C., Wade, S. L., & Wolfe, C. R. (2008). Lessons learned: The effect of prior technology use on the web-based interventions. *Cyberpsychology and Behavior, 11*(2), 188–195.

Carney, J., & Porter, P. (2009). School reentry for children with acquired central nervous system injuries. *Developmental Disabilities, 15*, 152–158.

Carroll, L. J., Cassidy, J. D., Holm, L., Kraus, J. F., & Coronado, V. G. (2004). Methodological issues and research recommendations for mild traumatic brain injury: The WHO collaborating centre task force on mild traumatic brain injury. *Journal of Rehabilitation Medicine, 43*, 113–125.

Casey, B. J., Giedd, J. N., & Thomas, K. M. (2000). Structural and functional brain development and its relation to cognitive development. *Biological Psychology, 54*(1–3), 241–257.

Cassidy, J. D., Carroll, L. J., Peloso, P. M., Borg, J., von Holst, H., Holm, L., . . . Coronado, V. G. (2004). Incidence, risk factors and prevention of mild traumatic brain injury: Results of the WHO Collaborating Centre Task Force on Mild Traumatic Brain Injury. *Journal of Rehabilitation Medicine, Supplement, 43*, 28–60.

Catale, C., Marique, P., Closser, A., & Meulemans, T. (2009). Attentional and executive functioning following mild traumatic brain injury in children using the Test for Attentional Performance (TAP) battery. *Journal of Clinical & Experimental Neuropsychology, 31*(3), 331–338.

Catroppa, C., & Anderson, V. (1999a). Attentional skills in the acute phase following pediatric traumatic brain injury. *Child Neuropsychology, 5*(4), 251–264.

Catroppa, C., & Anderson, V. (1999b). Recovery of educational skills following paediatric traumatic brain injury. *Pediatric Rehabilitation, 3*(4), 167–175.

Catroppa, C., & Anderson, V. (2002). Recovery in memory function in the first year following TBI in children. *Brain Injury, 16*(5), 369–384.

Catroppa, C., & Anderson, V. (2003). Children's attentional skills 2 years post-traumatic brain injury. *Developmental Neuropsychology, 23*(3), 359–373.

Catroppa, C., & Anderson, V. (2004). Recovery and predictors of language skills two years following pediatric traumatic brain injury. *Brain & Language, 88*(1), 68–78.

Catroppa, C., & Anderson, V. (2005). A prospective study of the recovery of attention from acute to 2 years post pediatric traumatic brain injury. *Journal of the International Neuropsychological Society, 11*, 84–98.

Catroppa, C., & Anderson, V. (2007). Recovery in memory function, and its relationship to academic success, at 24 months following pediatric TBI. *Child Neuropsychology, 13*(3), 240–261.

Catroppa, C., & Anderson, V. (2008). Intervention approaches for executive dysfunction following brain injury in childhood. In V. Anderson, R. Jacobs, & P. Anderson (Eds.), *Executive functions and the frontal lobes: A lifespan perspective* (pp. 439–469). New York, NY: Taylor & Francis.

Catroppa, C., Anderson, V., Muscara, F., Morse, S., Haritou, F., Rosenfeld, J., Heinrich, L.M. (2009). Educational skills – Long-term outcome and predictors following pediatric traumatic brain injury. *Neuropsychological Rehabilitation, 19*(5), 716–732.

Catroppa, C., & Anderson, V. (2010). Pediatric TBI: Challenges for treatment and rehabilitation. In V. Anderson & K. O. Yeates (Eds.), *Pediatric traumatic brain injury: New frontiers in clinical and translational research* (pp. 192–206). Cambridge, UK: Cambridge University Press.

Catroppa, C., & Anderson, V. (2011). Pediatric traumatic brain injury (TBI): Overview. In M. R. Schoenberg & J. G. Scott (Eds.), *The little black book of neuropsychology: A syndrome-based approach* (pp. 765–786). New York, NY: Springer Science and Business Media.

Catroppa, C., Anderson, V., Godfrey, C., & Rosenfeld, J.V. (2011). Attentional skills 10 years post pediatric traumatic brain injury (TBI). *Brain Injury, 25*(9), 858–869.

Catroppa, C., Anderson, V. A., Morse, S. A., Haritou, F., & Rosenfeld, J. V. (2007). Children's attentional skills 5 years post-TBI. *Journal of Pediatric Psychology, 32*(3), 354–369.

Catroppa, C., Anderson, V., Morse, S., Haritou, F., & Rosenfeld, J. (2008). Outcome and predictors of functional recovery five years following pediatric traumatic brain injury (TBI). *Journal of Pediatric Psychology, 33*(7), 707–718.

Catroppa, C., Anderson, V., & Muscara, F. (2009). Rehabilitation of executive skills post childhood traumatic brain injury (TBI): A pilot intervention study. *Developmental Neurorehabilitation, 12*(5), 361–369.

Catroppa, C., Anderson, V. A., Muscara, F., Morse, S. A., Haritou, F., Rosenfeld, J. V., & Heinrich, L. M. (2009). Educational skills: Long-term outcome and predictors following paediatric traumatic brain injury. *Neuropsychological Rehabilitation, 19*(5), 716–732.

Catroppa, C., Godfrey, C., Rosenfeld, J. V., Hearps, S.S.J.C., & Anderson, V. A. (2012). Functional recovery ten years after pediatric traumatic brain injury: Outcomes and predictors. *Journal of Neurotrauma, 29*(16), 2539–2547.

Catroppa, C., Stone, S., Rosema, S., Soo, C., & Anderson, V. (2014). Preliminary efficacy of an attention and memory intervention post-childhood brain injury. Case study. *Brain Injury, 28*(2), 252–260.

Cattelani, R., Lombardi, F., Brianti, R., & Mazzucchi, A. (1998). Traumatic brain injury in childhood: Intellectual, behavioural and social outcome into adulthood. *Brain Injury, 12*(4), 283–296.

Chadwick, O., Rutter, M., Brown, G., Shaffer, D., & Traub, M. (1981). A prospective study of children with head injuries: II. Cognitive sequelae. *Psychological Medicine, 11*, 49–61.

Chapman, L. A., Wade, S. L., Walz, N. C., Taylor, H. G., Stancin, T., & Yeates, K. O. (2010). Clinically significant behavior problems during the initial 18 months following early childhood traumatic brain injury. *Rehabilitation Psychology, 55*, 48–57.

Chapman, S. B., Culhane, K. A., Levin, H. S., Harward, H., Mendelsohn, D., Ewing-Cobbs, L., . . . Bruce, D. (1992). Narrative discourse after closed head injury in children and adolescents. *Brain and Language, 43*(1), 42–65.

Chapman, S. B., Gamino, J. F., Cook, L. G., Hanten, G., Li, X., & Levin, H.S. (2006). Impaired discourse gist and working memory in children after brain injury. *Brain and Language, 97*(2), 178–188.

Chapman, S. B., McKinnon, L., Levin, H. S., Song, J., Meier, M. C., & Chiu, S. (2001). Longitudinal outcome of verbal discourse in children with traumatic brain injury: Three-year follow-up. *Journal of Head Trauma Rehabilitation, 16*(5), 441–455.

Chapman, S. B., Sparks, G., Levin, H. S., Dennis, M., Roncadin, C., Zhang, L., & Song, J. (2004). Discourse macrolevel processing after severe pediatric traumatic brain injury. *Developmental Neuropsychology, 25*(1–2), 37–60.

Chastain, C. A., Oyoyo, U., Zipperman, M., Joo, E., Ashwal, S., Shutter, L., . . . Tong, K. A. (2009). Predicting outcomes of traumatic brain injury by imaging modality and injury distribution. *Journal of Neurotrauma, 26*(8), 1183–1196.

Chaytor, N., Temkin, N., Machamer, J., & Dikmen, S. (2007). The ecological validity of neuropsychological assessment and the role of depressive symptoms in moderate to severe traumatic brain injury. *Journal of the International Neuropsychological Society, 13*(3), 377–385.

Chertkoff Walz, N., Cecil, K. M., Wade, S. L., & Michaud, L. J. (2008). Late proton magnetic resonance spectroscopy following traumatic brain injury during early childhood: Relationship with neurobehavioral outcomes. *Journal of Neurotrauma, 25*, 94–103.

Chevignard, M., Brooks, N., & Truelle, J. L. (2010). Community integration following severe childhood traumatic brain injury. *Current Opinion in Neurology, 23*(6), 695–700.

Chevignard, M., Servant, V., Mariller, A., Abada, G., Pradat-Diehl, P., & Laurent-Vannier, A. (2009). Assessment of executive functioning in children after TBI with a naturalistic open-ended task: A pilot study. *Developmental Neurorehabilitation, 12*(2), 76–91.

Chevignard, M., Toure, H., Brugel, D. G., Poirer, J., & Laurent-Vannier, A. (2010). A comprehensive model of care for rehabilitation of children with acquired brain injuries. *Child Care Health Development, 36*(1), 31–43.

Chew, E., & Zafonte, R. D. (2009). Pharmacological management of neurobehavioral disorders following traumatic brain injury—A state-of-the-art review. *Journal of Rehabilitation Research and Development, 46*(6), 851–878.

Chiaretti, A., Antonelli, A., Mastrangelo, A., Pezzotti, P., Tortorolo, L., Tosi, F., . . . Genovese, O. (2008). Interleukin-6 and nerve growth factor upregulation correlates with improved outcome in children with severe traumatic brain injury. *Journal of Neurotrauma, 25*(3), 225–234.

Choe, M. C., Babikian, T., DiFiori, J., Hovda, D. A., & Giza, C. (2012). A pediatric perspective on concussion pathophysiology. *Current Opinion in Pediatrics, 24*, 1–7.

Chu, Z., Wilde, E. A., Hunter, J.V., McCauley, S. R., Bigler, E. D., Troyanskaya, M., . . . Levine, H. S. (2010). Voxel-based analysis of diffusion tensor imaging in mild traumatic brain injury in adolescents. *American Journal of Neuroradiology, 31*(2), 340–346.

Cicerone, K., Levin, H., Malec, J., Stuss, D., & Whyte, J. (2006). Cognitive rehabilitation interventions for executive function: Moving from bench to bedside in patients with traumatic brain injury. *Journal of Cognitive Neuroscience, 18*(7), 1212–1222.

Cicerone, K., & Tupper, D. (1990). Neuropsychological rehabilitation: Treatment of errors in everyday function. In D. Tupper & K. Cicerone (Eds.), *The neuropsychology of everyday life: Issues in development and rehabilitation* (pp. 271–291). Boston, MA: Kluwer Academic Publishers.

Ciesielski, K. T., Lesnik, P. G., Savoy, R. L., Grant, E. P., & Ahlfors, S. P. (2006). Developmental neural networks in children performing a Categorical N-Back Task. *Neuroimage, 33*(3), 980–990.

Clarke, L. A., Genat, R. C., & Anderson, J.F.I. (2012). Long-term cognitive complaint and post-concussive symptoms following mild traumatic brain injury: The role of cognitive and affective factors. *Brain Injury, 26*(3), 298–307.

Clifton, G. L. (2004). Is keeping cool still hot? An update on hypothermia in brain injury. *Current Opinion in Critical Care, 10*, 116–119.

Cloots, R., van Dommelen, J., Nyberg, T., Lleiven, S., & Geers. M. (2011). Micromechanics of diffuse axonal injury: Influence of axonal orientation and anisotropy. *Biotech Model Mechanobiol, 10*(3), 413–422.

Coats, B., & Margulies, S. S. (2006). Material properties of human infant skull and suture at high rates. *Journal of Neurotrauma, 23*, 1222–1232.

Colbert, C. A., Holshouser, B. A., Aaen, G. S., Sheridan, C., Oyoyo, U., Kido, D., . . . Ashwal, S. (2010). Value of cerebral microhemorrhages detected with susceptibility-weighted MR imaging for prediction of long-term outcome in children with nonaccidental trauma. *Radiology, 256*(3), 898–905.

Cole, W. R., Paulos, S. K., Cole, C. A. S., & Tankard, C. (2009). A review of family intervention guidelines for pediatric acquired brain injuries. *Developmental Disabilities, 15*, 159–166.

Coles, J. P. (2007). Imaging after brain injury. *British Journal of Anaesthesia, 99*(1), 49–60.

Collie, A., Maruff, P., Makdissi, M., McCrory, P., McStephen, M., & Darby, D. (2003). Cog-Sport: Reliability and correlation with conventional cognitive tests used in postconcussion medical evaluations. *Clin J Sport Med, 13*, 28–32.

Committee on Quality Improvement, American Academy of Pediatrics Commission on Clinical Policies and Research, American Academy of Family Physicians. (1999). The management of minor closed head injury in children. *Pediatrics, 104*, 1407–1415.

Conklin, H. M., Salorio, C. F., & Slomine, B. S. (2008). Working memory performance following paediatric traumatic brain injury. *Brain Injury, 22*(11), 847–857.

Conners, C. K., Sitarenios, G., Parker, J. D., & Epstein, J. N. (1998). The revised Conners' Parent Rating Scale (CPRS-R): Factor structure, reliability, and criterion validity. *Journal of Abnormal Child Psychology, 26*(4), 257–268.

Conners, G. P., Sacks, W. K., & Leahey, N. F. (1999). Variations in sedating uncooperative, stable children for post-traumatic head CT. *Pediatric Emergency Care, 15*(4), 241–244.

Cooper, D. J., Rosenfeld, J.V., Murray, L., Arabi,Y., Davies, A. R., D'Urso, P., . . . Wolfe, R. (2013). Decompressive craniectomy in diffuse traumatic brain injury. *New England Journal of Medicine, 364*, 1493–1502.

Cooper, J. D., Rosenfeld, J.V., & Wolfe, R. (2012). DECRA investigators response to "The future of decompressive craniectomy for diffuse traumatic brain injury" by Honeybul et al. *Journal of Neurotrauma, 29*, 2595–2596.

Copes, W. S., Sacco, W. J., Champion, H. R., & Bain, L. W. (1989). Progress in characterising anatomic injury. In *Proceedings of the 33rd Annual Meeting of the Association for the Advancement of Automotive Medicine, Baltimore, MD,* 205–218.

Corrigan, J. D., Lineberry, L. A., Komaroff, E., Langlois, J. A., Selassie, A. W., & Wood, K. D. (2007). Employment after traumatic brain injury: Differences between men and women. *Archives of Physical and Medical Rehabilitation, 88*, 1400–1409.

Coster, W. J., Haley, S., & Baryza, M. J. (1994). Functional performance of young children after traumatic brain injury: A 6-month follow-up study. *The American Journal of Occupational Therapy, 48*(3), 211–218.

Cowan, N. (1995). *Attention and memory: An integrated framework.* New York, NY: Oxford University Press.

Crepeau, F., & Scherzer, P. (1993). Predictors and indicators of work status after traumatic brain injury: A meta-analysis. *Neuropsychological Rehabilitation, 3*(1), 5–35.

Crichton, A., Knight, S., Oakley, E., Babl, F. E., & Anderson, V. (2015, Epub 2015 Mar 23). Fatigue in child chronic health conditions: A systematic review of assessment instruments. *Pediatrics, 135*(4), e1015–e1031.

Cronin, A. F. (2001). Traumatic brain injury in children: Issues in community function. *American Journal of Occupational Therapy, 55*, 377–384.

Crowe, L., Anderson, V., & Babl, F. E. (2010). Application of the CHALICE Clinical Prediction Rule for Intracranial Injury in Children outside the United Kingdom: Impact on head CT rate. *Archives of Disease in Childhood, 95*(12), 1017–1022.

Crowe, L., Babl, F., Anderson, V., & Catroppa, C. (2009). The epidemiology of paediatric head injuries: Data from a referral centre in Victoria, Australia. *Journal of Paediatrics & Child Health, 45*(6), 346–350.

Crowley, J. A., & Miles, M. A. (1991). Cognitive remediation in pediatric head injury: A case study. *Journal of Pediatric Psychology, 16*(5), 611–627.

Crowther, J. E., Hanten, G., Li, G., Dennis, M., Chapman, S. B., & Levin, H. S. (2011). Impairments in learning, memory, and metamemory following childhood head injury. *Journal of Head Trauma Rehabilitation, 26*(3), 192–201.

Cusick, A., McIntyre, S., Novack, I., Lannin, N., & Lowe, K. (2006). A comparison of goal attainment scaling and the Canadian occupational performance measure for paediatric rehabilitation research. *Developmental Neurorehabilitation, 9*(2), 149–157.

Dalby, P. R., & Obrzut, J. E. (1991). Epidemiologic characteristics and sequelae of closed head-injured children and adolescents: A review. *Developmental Neuropsychology, 7*, 35–68.

Dardiotis, E., Fountas, K. N., Dardioti, M., Xiromerisiou, G., Kapsalaki, E., Tasiou, A., . . . Hadjigeorgiou, G. M. (2010). Genetic association studies in patients with traumatic brain injury. *Neurosurgery Focus, 28*(1), 1–12.

Davis, M. J., & Vogel, L. (1995). Neurological assessment of the child with head trauma. *Journal of Dentistry for Children, 62*, 93–96.

Dawson, P., & Guare, R. (2004). *Executive skills in children and adolescents: A practical guide to assessment and intervention.* New York, NY: Guilford Press.

de Amorim e Silva, C. J., Mackenzie, A., Hallowell, L. M., Stewart, S. E., & Ditchfield, M. R. (2006). Practice MRI: Reducing the need for sedation and general anaesthesia in children undergoing MRI. *Australasian Radiology, 50*(4), 319–323.

de Bie, H. M., Boersma, M., Wattjes, M. P., Adriaanse, S., Vermeulen, R. J., Oostrom, K. J., . . . Delemarre-Van de Waal, H. A. (2010). Preparing children with a mock scanner training protocol results in high quality structural and functional MRI scans. *European Journal of Pediatrics, 169*(9), 1079–1085.

DeCuypere, M., & Klimo, P. (2012). Spectrum of traumatic brain injury from mild to severe. *Surgical Clinics North America, 92*, 939–957.

Degeneffe, C. E., Boot, D., Kuehne, J., Kuraishi, A., Maristela, F.-D., Noyes, J., . . . Will, H. (2008). Community-based interventions for persons with traumatic brain injury: A primer for rehabilitations counselors. *Journal of Applied Rehabilitation Counseling, 39*(1), 42–52.

Dennis, M. (1989). Language and the young damaged brain. In T. Boll & B. Bryant (Eds.), *Clinical neuropsychology and brain function: Research, measurement and practice* (pp. 89–123). Washington, DC: American Psychological Association.

Dennis, M., Agostino, A., Taylor, H. G., Bigler, E. D., Rubin, K., Vannatta, K., . . . Stancin, T. (2013). Emotion expression and socially modulated emotive communication in children with traumatic brain injury. *Journal of the International Neuropsychological Society, 18*, 1–10.

Dennis, M., & Barnes, M. A. (1990). Knowing the meaning, getting the point, bridging the gap and carrying the message: Aspects of discourse following closed head injury in childhood and adolescence. *Brain and Language, 39*, 428–446.

Dennis, M., Barnes, M. A., Donnelly, R. E., Wilkinson, M., & Humphreys, R. P. (1996). Appraising and managing knowledge: Metacognitive skills after childhood head injury. *Developmental Neuropsychology, 12*(1), 77–103.

Dennis, M., Guger, S., Roncadin, C., Barnes, M., & Schachar, R. (2001). Attentional-inhibitory control and social-behavioral regulation after childhood closed head injury: Do biological, developmental and recovery variables predict outcome? *Journal of the International Neuropsychological Society, 7*(6), 683–692.

Dennis, M., Simic, N., Taylor, H. G., Bigler, E. D., Rubin, K. H., Vannatta, K., . . . Yeates, K. O. (2012). Theory of mind in children with traumatic brain injury. *Journal of the International Neuropsychological Society, 18*, 908–916.

Dennis, M., Wilkinson, M., Koski, L., & Humphreys, R. P. (1995). Attention deficits in the long term after childhood head injury. In S. H. Broman & M. E. Michel (Eds.), *Traumatic head injury in children* (pp. 165–187). New York, NY: Oxford University Press.

Derogatos, L. (1994). *Symptom Checklist Revised.* Pearson Publications.

Di Battista, A., Godfrey, C., Soo, C., Catroppa, C., & Anderson, V. (2014). Depression and health related quality of life in adolescent survivors of a traumatic brain injury: A pilot study. *PLoS One, 9*(7).

Di Battista, A., Soo, C., Catroppa, C., & Anderson, V. (2012). Quality of life in children and adolescents post-TBI: A systematic review and meta-analysis. *Journal of Neurotrauma, 29*(9), 1717–1727.

Didus, E., Anderson, V., & Catroppa, C. (1999). The development of pragmatic communication skills in head injured children. *Pediatric Rehabilitation, 3*(4), 177–186.

Diedler, J., Sykora, M., Blatow, M., Juttler, E., Unterberg, A., & Hacke, W. (2009). Decompressive surgery for severe brain edema. *Journal of Intensive Care Medicine, 24*, 168–178.

Dijkers, M. P. (2004). Quality of life after traumatic brain injury: A review of research approaches and findings. *Archives of Physical and Medical Rehabilitation, 85*(2), 21–35.

Dikmen, S., Machamer, J., Winn, H., & Temkin, N. (1995). Neuropsychological outcome at 1-year post head injury. *Neuropsychology, 9*, 80–90.

DiScala, C. (1993). *National Pediatric Trauma Registry Biannual Report*, Phase 2.

Dise-Lewis, J. E., Lewis, H. C., & Reichardt, C. S. (2009). BrainSTARS: Pilot data on a team-based intervention program for students who have acquired brain injury. *Journal of Head Trauma Rehabilitation, 24*(3), 166–177.

Donders, J. (1993). Memory functioning after traumatic brain injury in children. *Brain Injury, 7*(5), 431–437.

Donders, J., & Warschausky, S. (2007). Neurobehavioral outcomes after early versus late childhood traumatic brain injury. *Journal of Head Trauma Rehabilitation, 22*(5), 296–302.

Dooley, J. J., Anderson, V., Hemphill, S. A., & Ohan, J. (2008). Aggression after pediatric traumatic brain injury: A theoretical approach. *Brain Injury, 22*(11), 836–846.

Draper, K., Ponsford, J., & Schonberger, M. (2007). Psychosocial and emotional outcomes 10 years following traumatic brain injury. *Journal of Head Trauma Rehabilitation, 22*(5), 278–287.

Ducreux, D., Huynh, I., Fillard, P., Renoux, J., Petit-Lacour, M. C., Marsot-Dupuch, K., . . . Lasjaunias, P. (2005). Brain MR diffusion tensor imaging and fibre tracking to differentiate between two diffuse axonal injuries. *Neuroradiology, 47*(8), 604–608.

Duhaime, A. C., Gean, A. D., Haacke, E. M., Hicks, R., Wintermark, M., Mukherjee, P., . . . Riedy, G. (2010). Common data elements in radiologic imaging of traumatic brain injury. *Archives of Physical Medicine and Rehabilitation, 91*(11), 1661–1666.

Duhaime, A., Gennarelli, T., Thibault, L., Bruce, D., Margulies, S., & Wiser, R. (1987). The shaken baby syndrome. A clinical, pathological, and biomechanical study. *Journal of Neurosurgery, 66*(3), 409–415.

Dumas, H. M., Haley, S. M., Carey, T. M., & Shen, P. (2004). The relationship between functional mobility and the intensity of physical therapy intervention in children with traumatic brain injury. *Pediatric Physical Therapy, 16*, 157–164.

Dunning, J., Daly, J. P., Lomas, J. P., Lecky, F., Batchelor, J., & Mackway-Jones, K. (2006). Derivation of the children's head injury algorithm for the prediction of important clinical events decision rule for head injury in children. *Archives of Disease in Childhood, 91*(11), 885–891.

Dykeman, B. F. (2003). School-based interventions for treating social adjustment difficulties in children with traumatic brain injury. *Journal of Instructional Psychology, 30*(3), 225–230.

Elliott, C. D. (2007). *Differential Ability Scales–Second Edition: Introductory and technical handbook.* San Antonio, TX: Psychological Corporation.

Elson, L., & Ward, C. (1994). Mechanisms and pathophysiology of mild head injury. *Seminars in Neurology, 14*, 8–18.

Emanuelson, I., & Uvebrant, P. (2009). Occurrence of epilepsy during the first 10 years after traumatic brain injury acquired in childhood up to the age of 18 years in the south western Swedish population-based series. *Brain Injury, 23*(7), 612–616.

Emanuelson, I. M., von Wendt, L., Bjure, J., Wiklund, L. M., & Uvebrant, P. (1997). Computed tomography and single-photon emission computed tomography as diagnostic tools in acquired brain injury among children and adolescents. *Developmental Medicine and Child Neurology, 39*(8), 502–507.

Engberg, A., & Teasdale, G. (2004). Psychosocial outcome following traumatic brain injury in adults: A long-term population-based follow-up. *Brain Injury, 18*(6), 533–545.

Epstein, J. N., Casey, B. J., Tonev, S. T., Davidson, M., Reiss, A. L., Garrett, A., . . . Spicer, J. (2007). Assessment and prevention of head motion during imaging of patients with attention deficit hyperactivity disorder. *Psychiatry Research, 155*(1), 75–82.

Erickson, S. J., Montague, E. Q., & Gerstle, M. A. (2010). Health-related quality of life in children with moderate-to-severe traumatic brain injury. *Developmental Neurorehabilitation, 13*(3), 175–181.

Ettenhofer, M. L., & Abeles, N. (2009). The significance of mild traumatic brain injury to cognition and self-reported symptoms in long-term recovery from injury. *Journal of Clinical & Experimental Neuropsychology, 31*(3), 363–372.

Evans, R. (1992). The postconcussion syndrome and the sequelae of mild head injury. *The Neurology of Trauma, 10,* 815–847.

Ewing-Cobbs, L., Barnes, M., Fletcher, J. M., Levin, H. S., Swank, P. R., & Song, J. (2004). Modeling of longitudinal academic achievement scores after pediatric traumatic brain injury. *Developmental Neuropsychology, 25*(1–2), 107–133.

Ewing-Cobbs, L., Brookshire, B., Scott, M. A., & Fletcher, J. M. (1998). Children's narratives following traumatic brain injury: Linguistic structure, cohesion and thematic recall. *Brain and Language, 61,* 395–419.

Ewing-Cobbs, L., & Fletcher, J. M. (1987). Neuropsychological assessment of head injury in children. *Journal of Learning Disabilities, 20*(9), 526–535.

Ewing-Cobbs, L., Levin, H. S., Eisenberg, H. M., & Fletcher, J. M. (1987). Language functions following closed-head injury in children and adolescents. *Journal of Clinical and Experimental Neuropsychology, 9*(5), 575–592.

Ewing-Cobbs, L., Levin, H. S., Fletcher, J. M., Miner, M. E., & Eisenberg, H. M. (1990). The children's orientation and amnesia test: Relationship to severity of acute head injury and to recovery of memory. *Neurosurgery, 27*(5), 683–691; discussion 691.

Ewing-Cobbs, L., Prasad, M., Kramer, L., Louis, P. T., Baumgartner, J., & Fletcher, J. M. (2000). Acute neuroradiologic findings in young children with inflicted or noninflicted traumatic brain injury. *Child's Nervous System, 16*(1), 25–33; discussion 34.

Ewing-Cobbs, L., Prasad, M. R., Kramer, L., Cox, C. S., Jr., Baumgartner, J., Fletcher, S. . . . Swank, P. (2006). Late intellectual and academic outcomes following traumatic brain injury sustained during early childhood. *Journal of Neurosurgery, 105*(4 Suppl), 287–296.

Ewing-Cobbs, L., Prasad, M. R., Swank, P., Kramer, L., Mendez, D., Treble, A., . . . Bachevalier, J. (2012). Social communication in young children with traumatic brain injury: Relations with corpus callosum morphometry. *International Journal of Developmental Neuroscience 30*(3), 247–254.

Ewing-Cobbs, L., Prasad, M. R., Swank, P., Kramer, L., Cox, C. S. Jr., Fletcher, J. M., . . . Hasan, K. M. (2008). Arrested development and disrupted callosal microstructure following pediatric traumatic brain injury: Relation to neurobehavioral outcomes. *Neuroimage, 42,* 1305–1315.

Fadyl, J. K., & McPherson, K. M. (2009). Approaches to vocational rehabilitation after traumatic brain injury: A review of the evidence. *Journal of Head Trauma Rehabilitation, 24*(3), 195–212.

Farkas, O., & Povlishock, J. T. (2007). Cellular and subcellular change evoked by diffuse traumatic brain injury: A complex web of change extending far beyond focal damage. *Progress in Brain Research, 161,* 43–59.

Farmer, J. E., Haut, J. S., Williams, J., Kapila, C., Johnstone, B., & Kirk, K. S. (1999). Comprehensive assessment of memory functioning following traumatic brain injury in children. *Developmental Neuropsychology, 15*(2), 269–289.

Farmer, J., Kanne, S., Haut, J., Williams, J., Johnstone, B., & Kirk, K. (2002). Memory functioning following traumatic brain injury in children with premorbid learning problems. *Developmental Neuropsychology, 22*(2), 455–469.

Fay, T. B., Yeates, K. O., Taylor, H. G., Bangert, B., Dietrich, A., Nuss, K. E., . . . Wright, M. (2009). Cognitive reserve as a moderator of postconcussive symptoms in children with complicated and uncomplicated mild traumatic brain injury. *Journal of the International Neuropsychological Society, 16,* 94–105.

Fay, G., Yeates, K. O., Wade, S. L., Drotar, D., Stancin, T., & Taylor, H. G. (2009). Predicting longitudinal patterns of functional deficits in children with traumatic brain injury. *Neuropsychology, 23*(3), 271–282.

Feeney, T. J., & Ylvisaker, M. (2003). Context-sensitive behavioural supports for young children with TBI. Short-term effects and long-term outcome. *Journal of Head Trauma and Rehabilitation, 18*(1), 33–51.

Feng, Y., Abney, T., Okamoto, R., Pless, R., Genin, G., & Bayly, P. (2010). Relative brain displacement and deformation during constrained mild frontal head impact. *J R Soc Interface, 6;7*(53), 1677–1688.

Fennell, E. B., & Mickle, J. P. (1992). Behavioural effects of head trauma in children and adolescents. In M. G. Tramontana & S. R. Hooper (Eds.), *Advances in child neuropsychology— Volume 1.* New York, NY: Springer-Verlag.

Field, M., Collins, M. W., Lovell, M. R., & Maroon, J. (2003). Does age play a role in recovery from sports-related concussion? A comparison of high school and collegiate athletes. *Journal of Pediatrics, 142,* 546–553.

Finkelstein, E. A., Corso, P. S., Miller, T. R., & Associates. (2006). *The incidence and economic burden of injuries in the United States.* New York, NY: Oxford University Press.

Fixsen, D., Naoom, S., Blase, K., Friedman, R., & Wallace, F. (2005). *Implementation research: A synthesis of the literature.* Tampa, FL: University of South Florida, Louis de la Parte Florida Mental Health Institute, The National Implementation Research Network, (FMHI Publication #231).

Flanagan, S. R. (2009). Managing agitation associated with traumatic brain injury: Behavioral versus pharmacologic interventions. *American Academy of Physical Medicine and Rehabilitation, 1,* 76–80.

Fletcher, J. M., Ewing-Cobbs, L., Francis, D. J., & Levin, H. S. (1995). Variability in outcomes after traumatic brain injury in children: A developmental perspective. In S. H. Broman & M. E. Michel (Eds.), *Traumatic head injury in children* (pp. 3–21). New York, NY: Oxford University Press.

Fletcher, J. M., Ewing-Cobbs, L., Miner, M. E., Levin, H. S., & Eisenberg, H. (1990). Behavioral changes after closed head injury in children. *Journal of Consulting and Clinical Psychology, 58*(1), 93–98.

Folkersma, H., Boellaard, R., Yaqub, M., Kloet, R. W., Windhorst, A. D., Lammertsma, A. A., . . . van Berckel, V. N. (2011). Widespread and prolonged increase in (R)-(11)C-PK11195 binding after traumatic brain injury. *Journal of Nuclear Medicine, 52*(8), 1235–1239.

Fraas, M., & Bellerose, A. (2010). Mentoring programme for adolescent survivors of acquired brain injury. *Brain Injury, 24*(1), 50–61.

Freilich, E. R., & Gaillard, W. D. (2010). Utility of functional MRI in pediatric neurology. *Curr Neurol Neurosci Rep, 10*(1), 40–46.

Fundaro, C., Caldarelli, M., Monaco, S., Cota, F., Giorgio, V., Filoni, S., . . . Onesimo, R. (2012). Brain CT for pediatric minor accidental head injury. An Italian experience and review of literature. *Child's Nervous System, 28*(7), 1063–1068.

Gabbe, B. J., Simpson, P. M., Sutherland, A. M., Palmer, C. S., Butt, W., Bevan, C., . . . Cameron, P. A. (2010). Agreement between parent and child report on health-related quality of life: Impact of time post-injury. *The Journal of Trauma, 69*(6), 1578–1582.

Gabbe, B. J., Simpson, P. M., Sutherland, A. M., Palmer, C. S., Butt, W., Bevan, C., . . . Cameron, P. (2011). Functional and health-related quality of life outcomes after pediatric trauma. *The Journal of Trauma, 70*(6), 1532–1538.

Gabriel, E. J., Ghajar, J., Jagoda, A., . . . Walters, B. C. (2002). Brain Trauma Foundation. Guidelines for Prehospital Management of Traumatic Brain Injury. *Journal of Neurotrauma, 19,* 111–174.

Gaetz, M. (2004). The neurophysiology of brain injury. *Clinical Neurophysiology, 115,* 4–18.

Gagner, C., Landry-Roy, C., Lainé, F., & Beauchamp, M. H. (2015). Apr 19, Epub ahead of print. Sleep-wake disturbances and fatigue after pediatric traumatic brain injury: A systematic review of the literature. *Journal of Neurotrauma.*

Gagnon, I., Galli, C., Friedman, D., Grilli, L., & Iverson, G. L. (2009). Active rehabilitation for children who are slow to recover following sport-related concussion. *Brain Injury, 23*(12), 956–964.

Galbiati, S., Recla, M., Pastore, V., Liscio, M., Bardoni, A., Castelli, E., . . . Strazzer, S. (2009). Attention remediation following traumatic brain injury in childhood and adolescence. *Neuropsychology, 23*(1), 40–49.

Gale, S. D., & Prigatano, G. P. (2010). Deep white matter volume loss and social reintegration after traumatic brain injury in children. *Journal of Head Trauma Rehabilitation, 25*(1), 15–22.

Gallagher, C. N., Hutchinson, P. J., & Pickard, J. D. (2007). Neuroimaging in trauma. *Current Opinion in Neurology, 20*(4), 403–409.

Galloway, N. R., Tong, K. A., Ashwal, S., Oyoyo, U., & Obenaus, A. (2008). Diffusion-weighted imaging improves outcome prediction in pediatric traumatic brain injury. *Journal of Neurotrauma, 25,* 1153–1162.

Galvin, J., McDonald, R., Catroppa, C., & Anderson, V. (2011). Does intervention using virtual reality improve upper limb function in children with neurological impairment: A systematic review of the evidence. *Brain Injury, 25*(5), 435–442.

Ganesalingam, K., Sanson, A., Anderson, V., & Yeates, K. O. (2006). Self-regulation and social and behavioral functioning following childhood traumatic brain injury. *Journal of the International Neuropsychological Society, 12*(5), 609–621.

Ganesalingam, K., Sanson, A., Anderson, V., & Yeates, K. O. (2007). Self-regulation as a mediator of the effects of childhood traumatic brain injury on social and behavioral functioning. *Journal of the International Neuropsychological Society, 13*(2), 298–311.

Ganesalingam, K., Yeates, K. O., Taylor, H. G., Chertkoff Walz, N., Stancin, T., & Wade, S. (2011). Executive functions and social competence in young children 6 months following traumatic brain injury. *Neuropsychology, 25*(4), 466–476.

Garnett, M. R., Blamire, A. M., Corkill, R. G., Cadoux-Hudson, T. A., Rajagopalan, B., & Styles, P. (2000). Early proton magnetic resonance spectroscopy in normal-appearing brain correlates with outcome in patients following traumatic brain injury. *Brain, 123*(10), 2046–2054.

Gavidia-Payne, S. T., & Hudson, A. (2002). Behavioural supports for parents of children with an intellectual disability and problem behaviours: An overview of the literature. *Journal of Intellectual and Developmental Disability, 27,* 31–55.

Gennarelli, T., & Thibault, L. (1982). Biomechanics of acute subdural hematoma. *Journal of Trauma, 22,* 680–686.

Gerrard-Morris, A., Taylor, H. G., Yeates, K. O., Walz, N. C., Stancin, T., Minich, N., . . . Wade, S. L. (2009). Cognitive development after traumatic brain injury in young children. *Journal of the International Neuropsychological Society, 16,* 157–168.

Gerring, J. P., Grados, M. A., Slomine, B., Christensen, J. R., Salorio, C. F., Cole, W. R., & Vasa, R. A. (2009). Disruptive behaviour disorders and disruptive symptoms after severe paediatric traumatic brain injury. *Brain Injury, 23,* 944–955.

Gerring, J. P., & Wade, S. (2012). The essential role of psychosocial risk and protective factors in pediatric traumatic brain injury research. *Journal of Neurotrauma, 29,* 621–628.

Gfroerer, S. D., Wade, S. L., & Wu, M. (2008). Parent perceptions of school-based support for students with traumatic brain injuries. *Brain Injury, 22*(9), 649–656.

Ghosh, A., Wilde, E. A., Hunter, J. V., Bigler, E. D., Chu, Z., Li, X., . . . Levin, H. S. (2009). The relation between Glasgow Coma Scale score and later cerebral atrophy in paediatric traumatic brain injury. *Brain Injury, 23*(3), 228–233.

Giedd, J. N., Blumenthal, J., Jeffries, N O., Castellanos, F. X., Liu, H., Zijdenbos, A., . . . Rapoport, J. L. (1999). Brain development during childhood and adolescence: A longitudinal MRI study. *Nature Neuroscience, 2*(10), 861–863.

Ginstfeldt, T., & Emanuelson, I. (2010). An overview of attention deficits after paediatric traumatic brain injury. *Brain Injury, 24*(10), 1123–1134.

Gioia, G. A., & Isquith, P. K. (2004). Ecological assessment of executive function in traumatic brain injury. *Developmental Neuropsychology, 25*(1–2), 135–158.

Gioia, G. A., Isquith, P. K., Guy, S. C., & Kenworthy, L. (2000). *Behavior Rating Inventory of Executive Function Professional Manual*. Odessa, FL: Psychological Assessment Resources.

Gioia, G., Schneider, J., Vaughn, C., & Isquith, P. (2009). Which symptom assessments and approaches are uniquely appropriate for paediatric concussion? *Br J Sports Med, 43*, i13–i22.

Giza, C. C., & Hovda, D. (2001). The neurometabolic cascade of concussion. *Journal of Athletic Training, 36*, 228–235.

Giza, C., Kutcher, J., Ashwal., S., Barth, J., Getchius, T., Gioia, G., . . . Zafonte, R. (2013). Summary of evidence-based guideline update: Evaluation and management of concussion in sports. *Neurology, 80*, 2250–2257.

Giza, C. C., Mink, R. B., & Madikians, A. (2007). Pediatric traumatic brain injury: Not just little adults. *Current Opinion in Critical Care, 13*, 143–152.

Giza, C. C., & Prins, M. L. (2006). Is being plastic fantastic? Mechanisms of altered plasticity after developmental traumatic brain injury. *Developmental Neuroscience, 28*(4–5), 364–379.

Glang, A., McLaughlin, K., & Schroeder, S. (2007). Using interactive multimedia to teach parent advocacy skills: An exploratory study. *Journal of Head Trauma Rehabilitation, 22*(3), 198–205.

Glang, A., Singer, G., Cooley, E., & Tish, N. (1992). Tailoring direct instruction techniques for use with elementary students with TBI. *Journal of Head Trauma Rehabilitation, 7*(4), 93–108.

Goldstein, F. C., & Levin, H. S. (1987). Epidemiology of pediatric closed head injury: Incidence, clinical characteristics and risk factors. *Journal of Learning Disabilities, 20*, 518–525.

Goldstein, F. C., & Levin, H. S. (1992). Cognitive function after closed head injury: Sequelae and outcome. In L. J. Thal, W. H. Moos, & E. R. Gamzu (Eds.), *Cognitive disorders: Pathophysiology and treatment* (pp. 61–92). New York, NY: Marcel Dekker.

Gomez-Perez, E., & Ostrosky-Solis, F. (2006). Attention and memory evaluation across the life span: Heterogeneous effects of age and education. *Journal of Clinical & Experimental Neuropsychology, 28*, 477–494.

Goodman, R. (1997). The Strengths and Difficulties Questionnaire: A research note. *J Child Psychol Psychiatry, 43*(9), 1159–1167.

Gordon, W. A., Zafonte, R., Cicerone, K., Cantor, J., Brown, M., Lombard, L., . . . Chandna, T. (2006). Traumatic brain injury rehabilitation. *American Journal of Physical Medicine & Rehabilitation, 85*, 343–382.

Goshen, E., Zwas, S. T., Shahar, E., & Tadmor, R. (1996). The role of 99Tcm-HMPAO brain SPET in paediatric traumatic brain injury. *Nuclear Medicine Communications, 17*(5), 418–422.

Gracey, F., Evans, J. J., & Malley, D. (2009). Capturing process and outcome in complex rehabilitation interventions: A "Y-shaped" model. *Neuropsychological Rehabilitation, 19*(6), 867–890.

Graham, J. R., Archer, R. P., Tellegen, A., Ben-Porath, Y. S., & Kaemmer, B. (2009). *Adolescent Minnesota Multiphasic Personality Inventory.* Pearson Publishing.

Gray, J., Robertson, I., Pentland, B., & Anderson, S. (1992). Microcomputer-based attentional retraining after brain damage: A randomised group controlled trial. *Neuropsychological Rehabilitations, 2*, 97–115.

Green, L., Godfrey, C., Soo, C., Anderson, V., & Catroppa, C. (2012). Agreement between parent-adolescent ratings on psychosocial outcome and quality-of-life following childhood traumatic brain injury. *Developmental Neurorehabilitation, 15*(2), 105–113.

Green, L. L., Godfrey, C., Soo, C., Anderson, V., & Catroppa, C. (2013). A preliminary investigation into psychosocial outcome and quality-of-life in adolescents following childhood Traumatic Brain Injury. *Brain Injury, 27*(7–8), 872–877.

Gronwall, D., Wrightson, P., & McGinn, V. (1997). Effect of mild head injury during the preschool years. *Journal of the International Neuropsychological Society, 3*, 592–597.

Grubenhoff, J. A., & Provance, A. (2012). Physical and neurological exam. In M. W. Kirkwood & K. O. Yeates (Eds.), *Mild traumatic brain injury in children and adolescents: From basic science to clinical management* (pp. 196–217). New York, NY: Guilford Press.

Gualtieri, C., & Johnson, L. (2006). Reliability and validity of a computerized neurocognitive test battery, CNS Vital Signs. *Arch Clin Neuropsychol, 21*(7), 623–643.

Guerguerian, A., Milly Lo, T. Y., & Hutchison, J. S. (2009). Clinical management and functional neuromonitoring in traumatic brain injury in children. *Current Opinion in Pediatrics, 21*(6), 737–744.

Guerin, F., Kennepohl, S., Leveille, G., Dominique, A., & McKerral, M. (2006). Vocational outcome indicators in atypically recovering mild TBI: A post-intervention study. *NeuroRehabilitation, 21*(4), 295–303.

Gurdin, L., Huber, S., & Cochran, C. (2005). A critical analysis of data-based studies examining behavioral interventions with children and adolescents with brain injury. *Behavioral Interventions, 20*, 3–16.

Guskiewicz, K., & Mihalik, J. (2011). Biomechanics of sport concussion: Quest for the elusive injury threshold. *Exercise Sports Science Review, 39*, 411.

Guskiewicz, K. K., Ross, S. E., & Marshall, S. W. (2001). Postural stability and neuropsychological deficits after concussion in collegiate athletes. *Journal of Athletic Training, 36*, 263–273.

Haacke, E. M., Duhaime, A. C., Gean, A. D., Riedy, G., Wintermark, M., Mukherjee, P., . . . Smith, D. H. (2010). Common data elements in radiologic imaging of traumatic brain injury. *Journal of Magnetic Resonance Imaging, 32*(3), 516–543.

Haacke, E. M., Xu, Y., Cheng, Y. C., & Reichenbach, J. R. (2004). Susceptibility weighted imaging (SWI). *Magn Reson Med, 52*(3), 612–618.

Hagen, C. (1998). *The Rancho levels of cognitive functioning.* Encinitas, CA: Rancho Los Amigos Medical Center.

Haitsma, I. K., & Maas, A. I. (2007). Monitoring cerebral oxygenation in traumatic brain injury. *Progress in Brain Research, 161*, 207–216.

Haley, S. M., Coster, W. J., Ludlow, L. H., Haltiwanger, J. T., & Andrellos, P. J. (1999). *The Pediatric Evaluation of Disability Inventory.* San Antonio, TX: The Psychological Corporation.

Hall, E. J. (2002). Lessons we have learned from our children: Cancer risks from diagnostic radiology. *Pediatric Radiology, 32*(10), 700–706.

Hallett, T. L. (1997). Linguistic competence in paediatric closed head injury. *Pediatric Rehabilitation, 1*(4), 219–228.

Halstead, M. E., & Walter, K. D. (2010). American Academy of Pediatrics. Clinical report—sport-related concussion in children and adolescents. *Pediatrics, 126*, 597–615.

Hamilton, N. A., & Keller, M. S. (2010). Mild traumatic brain injury in children. *Seminars in Pediatric Surgery, 19*, 271–278.

Hanten, G., Bartha, M., & Levin, H. S. (2000). Metacognition following pediatric traumatic brain injury: A preliminary study. *Developmental Neuropsychology, 18*(3), 383–398.

Hanten, G., Cook, L., Orsten, K., Chapman, S. B., Li, X., Wilde, E. A., . . . Levin, H. S. (2011). Effects of traumatic brain injury on a virtual reality social problem solving task and relations to cortical thickness in adolescence. *Neuropsychologia, 49*(3), 486–497.

Hanten, G., Dennis, M., Zhang, L., Barnes, M., Roberson, G., Archibald, J., . . . Levin, H. S. (2004). Childhood head injury and metacognitive processes in language and memory. *Developmental Neuropsychology, 25*(1–2), 85–106.

Hanten, G., Levin, H. S., & Song, J. X. (1999). Working memory and metacognition in sentence comprehension by severely head-injured children: A preliminary study. *Developmental Neuropsychology, 16*(3), 393–414.

Hanten, G., Scheibel, R., Li, X., Oomer, L., Stallings-Robertson, G., Hunter, V., . . . Levin, H. S. (2006). Decision making after traumatic brain injury in children. *Neurocase, 12*, 247–251.

Hanten, G., Wilde, E. A., Menefee, D. S., Li, X., Lane, S., Vasquez, C., . . . Levin, H. S. (2008). Correlates of social problem solving during the first year after traumatic brain injury in children. *Neuropsychology, 22*(3), 357–370.

Haque, A., & Enam, A. (2009). Implementation of Brain Trauma Foundation guidelines in children with acute traumatic brain injury in tertiary-care hospital in Pakistan. *Indian Journal of Neurotrauma, 6*, 111–114.

Hardman, J., & Manoukian, A. (2002). Pathology of head trauma. *Neuroimaging Clinics North America, 12*, 175–187.

Harris, E., Schuerholz, L., Singer, H., Reader, M., Brown, J., Cox, C., . . . Denckla, M. (1995). Executive function in children with Tourette's syndrome and/or attention deficit hyperactivity disorder. *Journal of the International Neuropsychological Society, 1*, 511–516.

Harris, J. R. (1996). Verbal rehearsal and memory in children with closed head injury: A quantitative and qualitative analysis. *Journal of Communication Disorders, 29*, 79–93.

Harrison, P. L., & Oakland, T. (2003). *Adaptive Behavior Assessment System—Second Edition.* San Antonio, TX: The Psychological Corporation.

Hart, T., Dijkers, M., Whyte, J., Braden, C., Trott, C. T., & Fraser, R. (2010). Vocational interventions and supports following job placement for persons with traumatic brain injury. *Journal of Vocational Rehabilitation, 32*, 135–150.

Hathaway, S., & McKinley, J. (1989). *MMPI-2 manual for administration and scoring.* Minneapolis, MN: University of Minnesota Press.

Hawley, C. A. (2004). Behaviour and school performance after brain injury. *Brain Injury, 18*(7), 645–659.

Hawley, C. A., Ward, A. B., Magnay, A. R., & Mychalkiw, W. (2004). Return to school after brain injury. *Archives of Disease in Childhood, 89*, 136–142.

Herman, S. T. (2002). Epilepsy after brain insult: Targeting epileptogenesis. *Neurology, 59*(9 Suppl 5), S21–26.

Hessen, E., Anderson, V., & Nestvold, K. (2008). MMPI-2 profiles 23 years after paediatric mild traumatic brain injury. *Brain Injury, 22*(1), 39–50.

Hessen, E., Nestvold, K., & Anderson, V. (2007). Neuropsychological function 23 years after mild traumatic brain injury: A comparison of outcome after paediatric and adult head injuries. *Brain Injury, 21*(9), 963–979.

Hibbard, M. R., Bogdany, J., Uysal, S., Kepler, K., Silver, J. M., Gordon, W. A., & Haddad, L. (2000). Axis II psychopathology in individuals with traumatic brain injury. *Brain Injury, 14*(1), 45–61.

High, W. M. Jr., Levin, H. S., & Gary, H. E. Jr. (1989). Recovery of orientation following closed head injury. *Journal of Clinical and Experimental Neuropsychology, 12,* 703–714.

Hillary, F. G., Slocomb, J., Hills, E. C., Fitzpatrick, N. M., Medaglia, J. D., Wang, J., . . . Wylie, G. R. (2011). Changes in resting connectivity during recovery from severe traumatic brain injury. *International Journal of Psychophysiology, 82*(1), 115–123.

Hillary, F. G., Steffener, J., Biswal, B. B., Lange, G., DeLuca, J., & Ashburner, J. (2002). Functional magnetic resonance imaging technology and traumatic brain injury rehabilitation: Guidelines for methodological and conceptual pitfalls. *Journal of Head Trauma Rehabilitation, 17*(5), 411–430.

Hodgson, J., McDonald, S., Tate, R., & Gertier, P. (2005). A randomised control trial of a cognitive-behavioural therapy program for managing social anxiety after acquired brain injury. *Brain Impairment, 6*(3), 69–180.

Holden, M. K. (2005). Virtual environments for motor rehabilitation: Review. *Cyberpsychology and Behavior, 8*(3), 187–211.

Holloway, M., Bye, A., & Moran, K. (1994). Non-accidental head injury in children. *The Medical Journal of Australia, 160,* 786–789.

Holmes, J. F., Borgialli, D. A., Nadel, F. M., Quayle, K. S., Schambam, N., Cooper, A., . . . Kuppermann, N. (2011). Do children with blunt head trauma and normal cranial computed tomography scan results require hospitalization for neurologic observation? *Annals of Emergency Medicine, 58,* 315–322.

Holshouser, B. A., Ashwal, S., Luh, G. Y., Shu, S., Kahlon, S., Auld, K. L., . . . Hinshaw, Jr., D. B. (1997). Proton MR spectroscopy after acute central nervous system injury: Outcome prediction in neonates, infants, and children. *Radiology, 202*(2), 487–496.

Holshouser, B. A., Tong, K. A., & Ashwal, S. (2005). Proton MR spectroscopic imaging depicts diffuse axonal injury in children with traumatic brain injury. *AJNR Am J Neuroradiol, 26*(5), 1276–1285.

Honeybul, S., Ho, K. M., Lind, C.R.P., & Gillett, G. R. (2011). The future of decompressive craniectomy for diffuse traumatic brain injury. *Journal of Neurotrauma, 28,* 2199–2200.

Hoofien, D., Gilboa, A., Vakil, E., & Donovick, P. J. (2001). Traumatic brain injury (TBI) 10–20 years later: A comprehensive outcome study of psychiatric symptomatology, cognitive abilities and psychosocial functioning. *Brain Injury, 15*(3), 189–209.

Hoofien, D., Vakil, E., Gilboa, A., Donovick, P. J., & Barak, O. (2002). Comparison of the predictive power of socio-economic variables, severity of injury and age on long-term outcome of traumatic brain injury: Sample-specific variables versus factors as predictors. *Brain Injury, 16*(1), 9–27.

Hooper, S. R., Alexander, J., Moore, D., Sasser, H. C., Laurent, S., King, J., . . . Callahan, B. (2004). Caregiver reports of common symptoms in children following a traumatic brain injury. *NeuroRehabilitation, 19,* 175–189.

Horneman, G., & Emanuelson, I. (2009). Cognitive outcome in children and young adults who sustained severe and moderate traumatic brain injury 10 years earlier. *Brain Injury, 23*(11), 907–914.

Hossain-Ibrahim, M. K., Tarnaris, A., & Wasserberg, J. (2012). Decompressive craniectomy—friend or foe? *Trauma, 14,* 16–38.

Hsiang, J.K., Chesnut, R.M., Crisp, C.B., Klauber, M. R., Blunt, B.A., & Marshall, L.F. (1994). Early, routine paralysis for intracranial pressure control in severe head injury: Is it necessary? *Critical Care Medicine, 22*, 1471–1476.

Huang, M.X., Theilmann, R. J., Robb, A., Angeles, A., Nichols, S., Drake, A., . . . Lee, R. R. (2009). Integrated imaging approach with MEG and DTI to detect mild traumatic brain injury in military and civilian patients. *Journal of Neurotrauma, 26*(8), 1213–1226.

Hudson, A., Matthews, J., Gavidia-Payne, S., Cameron, C., Mildon, R., & Radler, G. (2003). Evaluation of an intervention system for parents of children with intellectual disability and challenging behaviour. *Journal of Intellectual Disability Research, 47*, 238–249.

Hulka, F., Mullins, R. J., Mann, N. C., Hedges, J. R., Rowland, D., Worrall, W. H., . . . Trunkey, D. D. (1997). Influence of a statewide trauma system on pediatric hospitalization and outcome. *Journal of Trauma, 42*, 514–519.

Hunter, J.V., Thornton, R. J., Wang, Z. J., Levin, H. S., Roberson, G., Brooks, W. M., & Swank, P. R. (2005). Late proton MR spectroscopy in children after traumatic brain injury: Correlation with cognitive outcomes. *AJNR Am J Neuroradiol, 26*(3), 482–488.

Hunter, J.V., Wilde, E. A., Tong, K. A., & Holshouser, B. A. (2012). Emerging imaging tools for use with traumatic brain injury research. *Journal of Neurotrauma, 29*(4), 654–671.

Hutchison, J., Ward, R., Lacroix, J., Hébert, P., Skippen, P., Barnes, M., . . . Moher, D. for the HyP-HIT investigators and The Canadian Critical Care Trials Group. (2006). Hypothermia Pediatric Head Injury Trial (HyP-HIT): The value of a pre-trial clinical evaluation phase. *Developmental Neuroscience, 28*, 291–301.

Hutchison, J.S., Ward, R. E., Lacroix, J., Hébert, P. C., Barnes, M. A., Bohn, D. J., . . . Skippen, P. W. (2008). Hypothermia therapy after traumatic brain injury in children. *The New England Journal of Medicine, 358*, 2447–2456.

Hynd, G. W., & Willis, W. G. (Eds.). (1988). *Intercranial injuries. Paediatric neuropsychology.* New York, NY: Grune and Stratton, Inc.

Iverson, G. L., Brooks, B. L., Collins, M. W., & Lovell, M. R. (2006). Tracking neuropsychological recovery following concussion in sport. *Brain Injury, 20*(3), 245–252.

Iverson, G. L., Lange, R. T., Waljas, M., Liimatainen, S., Dastidar, P., Hartikainen, K. M., . . . Öhman, J. (2012). Outcome from complicated versus uncomplicated mild traumatic brain injury. *Rehabilitation Research and Practice.* doi:10.1155/2102/415740.

Jacobs, R., & Anderson, V. (2002). Planning and problem solving skills following focal frontal brain lesions in childhood: Analysis using the Tower of London. *Child Neuropsychology, 8*(2), 93–106.

Jaffe, K. M., Polissar, N. L., Fay, G. C., & Liao, S. (1995). Recovery trends over three years following pediatric traumatic brain injury. *Archives of Physical Medicine and Rehabilitation, 76*, 17–26.

Jagannathan, J., Okonkwo, D. O., Yeoh, H. K., Dumont, A. S., Saulle, D., Haizlip, J., . . . Jane, J. A. Jr. (2008). Long-term outcomes and prognostic factors in pediatric patients with severe traumatic brain injury and elevated intracranial pressure. *J Neurosurg Pediatr, 2*(4), 240–249.

Janusz, J. A., Kirkwood, M. W., Yeates, K. O., & Taylor, H. G. (2002). Social problem-solving skills in children with traumatic brain injury: Long-term outcomes and prediction of social competence. *Child Neuropsychology, 8*(3), 179–194.

Jennett, B., & Bond, M. (1975). Assessment of outcome after severe brain damage: A practical scale. *Lancet, 305*(7905), 480–484.

Jeremitski, E., Omert, L., Dunham, C., Wilberger, J., & Rodriguez, A. (2005). The impact of hyperglycemia on patients with severe brain injury. *Journal of Trauma, 58,* 47–50.

Jiang, J., & Yang, X. (2007). Current status of cerebral protection with mild-to-moderate hypothermia after traumatic brain injury. *Current Opinion in Critical Care, 13*, 153–155.

Johns, M. W. (1991). A new method for measuring daytime sleepiness: The Epworth sleepiness scale. *Sleep, 14*, 540–545.

Johnson, A. R., DeMatt, E., & Salorio, C. F. (2009). Predictors of outcome following acquired brain injury in children. *Developmental Disabilities, 15*, 124–132.

Johnson, D. L., & Krishnamurthy, S. (1996). Send severely head-injured children to a pediatric trauma center. *Pediatric Neurosurgery, 25*, 309–314.

Johnstone, B., Hexum, C. L., & Ashkanazi, G. (1995). Extent of cognitive decline in traumatic brain injury based on estimates of premorbid intelligence. *Brain Injury, 9*(4), 377–384.

Jonsson, C. A., Horneman, G., & Emanuelson, I. (2004). Neuropsychological progress during 14 years after severe traumatic brain injury in childhood and adolescence. *Brain Injury, 18*(9), 921–934.

Jonsson, C., & Elgmark Andersson, E. (2013). Mild traumatic brain injury: A description of how children and youths between 16 and 18 years of age perform leisure activities after 1 year. *Developmental Neurorehabilitation, 16*(1), 1–8.

Jordan, F. M., & Murdoch, B. E. (1994). Severe closed head injury in childhood: Linguistic outcomes into adulthood. *Brain Injury, 8*(6), 501–508.

Jordan, F. M., Murdoch, B. E., & Buttsworth, D. L. (1991). Closed-head-injured children's performance on narrative tasks. *Journal of Speech and Hearing Research, 34*, 572–582.

Josie, K. L., Peterson, C. C., Burant, C., Drotar, D., Stancin, T., Wade, S. L., . . . Taylor, H. G. (2008). Predicting family burden following childhood traumatic brain injury: A cumulative risk approach. *Journal of Head Trauma Rehabilitation, 23*(6), 357–368.

Kail, R. (1986). Sources of age differences in speed of processing. *Child Development, 57*, 969–987.

Kaldoja, M. L., & Kolk, A. (2012). Social-emotional behaviour in infants and toddlers with mild traumatic brain injury. *Brain Injury, 26*(7–8), 1005–1013.

Kamerling, S. N., Lutz, N., Posner, J. C., & Vanore, M. (2003). Mild traumatic brain injury in children: Practice guidelines for emergency department and hospitalized patients. *Pediatric Emergency Care, 19*, 431–440.

Karunanayaka, P. R., Holland, S. K., Yuan, W., Altaye, M., Jones, B. V., Michaud, L. J., . . . Wade, S. L. (2007). Neural substrate differences in language networks and associated language-related behavioral impairments in children with TBI: A preliminary fMRI investigation. *NeuroRehabilitation, 22*, 355–369.

Kasahara, M., Menon, D. K., Salmond, C. H., Outtrim, J. G., Taylor Tavares, J. V., Carpenter, T. A., . . . Stamatakis, E. A. (2010). Altered functional connectivity in the motor network after traumatic brain injury. *Neurology, 75*(2), 168–176.

Kaufmann, P. M., Fletcher, J. M., Levin, H. S., Miner, M. E., & Ewing-Cobbs, L. (1993). Attentional disturbance after pediatric closed head injury. *Journal of Child Neurology, 8*, 348–353.

Kazdin, A. E. (1984). *Behavior modification in applied settings*. Chicago, IL: The Dorsey Press.

Keenan, H., & Bratton, S. (2006). Epidemiology and outcomes of pediatric brain injury. *Developmental Neuroscience, 28*(4–5), 256–263.

Keenan, H., Runyan, D., Marshall, S., Nocera, M., Merton, D., & Sinal, S. (2003). A population based study of inflicted traumatic brain injury in young children. *JAMA, 290*, 621–626.

Keightley, M. L., Sinopoli, K. J., Davis, K. D., Mikulis, D. J., Wennberg, R., Tartaglia, M. C., . . . Tator, C. H. (2014). Is there evidence for neurodegenerative change following traumatic brain injury in children and youth? A scoping review. *Front Hum Neurosci, 8*, 139.

Kelly, J., & Rosenberg, J. (1997). Diagnosis and management of sports concussion. *Neurology, 48*, 575–580.

Kendall, E., Muenchberger, H., & Gee, T. (2006). Vocational rehabilitation following traumatic brain injury: A quantitative synthesis of outcome studies. *Journal of Vocational Rehabilitation, 25*, 149–160.

Kennard, M. (1936). Age and other factors in motor recovery from precentral lesions in monkeys. *American Journal of Physiology, 115*, 138–146.

Kenny, D. T., & Jennings, C. J. (2007). The relationship between head injury and violent offending in juvenile detainees. *Crime and Justice, 107*, 1–15.

Kim, E., Lauterbach, E. C., Reeve, A., Arciniegas, D. B., Coburn, K. L., Mendez, M. F., . . . Coffey, E. C. (2007). Neuropsychiatric complications of traumatic brain injury: A critical review (A report by the ANPA Committee on Research). *Journal of Neuropsychiatry and Clinical Neuroscience, 19*(2), 106–127.

Kim, J. J., & Gean, A. D. (2011). Imaging for the diagnosis and management of traumatic brain injury. *Neurotherapeutics: The Journal of the American Society for Experimental Neurotherapeutics, 8*, 39–53.

King, G. A., Law, M., King, S., Hurley, P., Hanna, S., Kertoy, M., & Rosenbaum, P. (2006). Measuring children's participation in recreation and leisure activities: Construct validation of the CAPE and PAC. *Child Care Health and Development, 33*(1), 38–39.

King, N., Crawford, S., Wenden, F., Moss, N., & Wade, D. (1995). The Rivermead Post Concussion Symptoms Questionnaire: A measure of symptoms commonly experienced after head injury and its reliability. *Journal of Neurology, 242*, 587–592.

Kinsella, G., Prior, M., Sawyer, M., Murtagh, D., Eisenmajer, R., Anderson, V., . . . Klug, G. (1995). Neuropsychological deficit and academic performance in children and adolescents following traumatic brain injury. *Journal of Pediatric Psychology, 20*, 753–767.

Kinsella, G., Prior, M., Sawyer, M., Ong, B., Murtagh, D., Eisenmajer, R., . . . Klug, G. (1997). Predictors and indicators of academic outcome in children 2 years following traumatic head injury. *Journal of the International Neuropsychological Society, 3*, 608–616.

Klonoff, H., Clark, C., & Klonoff, P. S. (1993). Long-term outcome of head injuries: A 23 year follow up study of children with head injuries. *Journal of Neurology, Neurosurgery and Psychiatry, 56*(4), 410–415.

Klonoff, P., & Lamb, D. (1996). Mild head injury, significant impairment on neuropsychological test scores, and psychiatric disability. *The Clinical Neuropsychologist, 12*, 31–42.

Kneafsey, R., & Gawthorpe, D. (2004). Head injury: Long-term consequences for patients and families and implications for nurses. *Neurology, 13*, 601–608.

Kochanek, P. M. (2005). Pediatric traumatic brain injury: Beyond the guidelines. *Current Treatment Options in Neurology, 7*, 441–450.

Kochanek, P. (2006). Pediatric traumatic brain injury: Quo vadis? *Developmental Neurosciemce, 28*, 244–255.

Kochanek, P. M., Carney, N., & Adelson, P. D. (2012). Guidelines for the acute medical management of severe traumatic brain injury in infants, children, and adolescents: Second Edition. *Pediatric Critical Care Medicine, 13*(Suppl. 1), 1–82.

Koelfen, W., Freund, M., Dinter, D., Schmidt, B., Koenig, S., Schultze, C., & Runde, J. (1997). Long-term follow up of children with head injuries-classified as "good recovery" using the Glasgow Outcome Scale: Neurological, neuropsychological and magnetic resonance imaging results. *European Journal of Pediatrics, 156*(3), 230–235.

Koepsell, T., Rivara, F., Vavilala, M., Wang, J., Temkin, N., Jaffe, K., & Durbin, D. (2011). Incidence and descriptive epidemiologic features of traumatic brain injury in King County, Washington. *Pediatrics, 128*(5), 946–954.

Kolb, B., & Gibb, R. (1999). Neuroplasticity and recovery of function after brain injury. In D. Stuss, G. Winocur, & I. Robertson (Eds.), *Cognitive neurorehabilitation* (pp. 9–25). New York, NY: Cambridge University Press.

Kolb, B., & Wishaw, Q. (1996). *Fundamentals of human neuropsychology.* New York, NY: W. H. Freeman.

Korkman, M., Kirk, U., & Kemp, S. (2007). *NEPSY-II: A Developmental Neuropsychological Assessment* (2nd ed.). San Antonio, TX: The Psychological Corporation.

Koskiniemi, M., Kyykka, T., Nybo, T., & Jarho, L. (1995). Long-term outcome after severe brain injury in preschoolers is worse than expected. *Archives of Pediatrics and Adolescent Medicine, 149*(3), 249–254.

Kotsoni, E., Byrd, D., & Casey, B. J. (2006). Special considerations for functional magnetic resonance imaging of pediatric populations. *J Magn Reson Imaging, 23*(6), 877–886.

Kou, Z., Wu, Z., Tong, K. A., Holshouser, B., Benson, R. R., Hu, J., . . . Haacke, E. M. (2010). The role of advanced MR imaging findings as biomarkers of traumatic brain injury. *Journal of Head Trauma Rehabilitation, 25*(4), 267–282.

Kramer, M. E., Chiu, C. Y., Walz, N. C., Holland, S. K., Yuan, W., Karunanayaka, P., & Wade, S. L. (2008). Long-term neural processing of attention following early childhood traumatic brain injury: fMRI and neurobehavioral outcomes. *Journal of the International Neuropsychological Society, 14*(3), 424–435.

Kraus, J. F. (1995). Epidemiological features of brain injury in children: Occurrence, children at risk, causes and manner of injury, severity, and outcomes. In S. H. Broman & M. E. Michel (Eds.), *Traumatic head injury in children* (pp. 22–39). New York, NY: Oxford University Press.

Kraus, J. F., Fife, D., Cox, P., Ramstein, K., & Conroy, C. (1986). Incidence, severity, and external causes of pediatric brain injury. *American Journal of Diseases of Children, 140*, 687–693.

Kreutzer, J. S., Stejskal, T. M., Ketchum, J. M., Matwitz, J. H., Taylor, L. A., & Menzel, J. C. (2009). A preliminary investigation of the brain injury family intervention: Impact on family members. *Brain Injury, 23*(6), 535–547.

Kuppermann, N., Holmes, J. F., Dayan, P. S., Hoyle, J. D., Jr., Atabaki, S. M., Holubkov, R., . . . Wooten-Gorges, S. L. (2009). Identification of children at very low risk of clinically-important brain injuries after head trauma: A prospective cohort study. *Lancet, 374*(9696), 1160–1170.

Kurowski, B., Wade, S. L., Cecil, K. M., Walz, N. C., Yuan, W., Rajagopal, A., & Holland, S. K. (2009). Correlation of diffusion tensor imaging with executive function measures after early childhood traumatic brain injury. *Journal of Pediatric Rehabilitation Medicine, 2*(4), 273–283.

Laatsch, L., Harrington, D., Hotz, G., Marcantuono, J., Mozzoni, M. P., Walsh, V., & Hersey, K. P. (2007). An evidence-based review of cognitive and behavioral rehabilitation treatment studies in children with acquired brain injury. *Journal of Head Trauma Rehabilitation, 22*(4), 248–256.

Lachapelle, J., Bolduc-Teasdale, J., Ptito, A., & McKerral, M. (2008). Deficits in complex visual information processing after mild TBI: Electrophysiological markers and vocational outcome prognosis. *Brain Injury, 22*(3), 265–274.

Lachar, D. (1992). *Personality Inventory for Children (Revised formal manual supplement).* Los Angeles, CA: Western Psychological Services.

Lah, S., Epps, A., Levick, W., & Parry, L. (2011). Implicit and explicit memory outcome in children who have sustained severe traumatic brain injury: Impact of age at injury (preliminary findings). *Brain Injury, 25*(1), 44–52.

Lajiness-O'Neill, R., Erdodi, L., & Bigler, E. D. (2010). Memory and learning in pediatric traumatic brain injury: A review and examination of moderators of outcome. *Applied Neuropsychology, 17*, 83–92.

Landis, J., Hanten, G., Levin, H. S., Li, X., Ewing-Cobbs, L., Duron, J., . . . High, W. M. Jr. (2006). Evaluation of the errorless learning technique in children with traumatic brain injury. *Archives of Physical and Medical Rehabilitation, 87*, 799–805.

Langlois, J. A., Rutland-Brown, W., & Thomas, K. E. (2006). *Traumatic brain injury in the United States: Emergency Department Visits, Hospitalizations, and Deaths.* Atlanta, GA: Centers for Disease Control and Prevention, National Center for Injury Prevention and Control.

Lawson, M. J., & Rice, D. N. (1989). Effects of training in use of executive strategies on a verbal memory problem resulting from closed head injury. *Journal of Clinical & Experimental Neuropsychology, 6*, 842–854.

Le, T. H., & Gean, A. D. (2009). Neuroimaging of traumatic brain injury. *Mount Sinai Journal of Medicine, 76*, 145–162.

Lee, H., Wintermark, M., Gean, A. D., Ghajar, J., Manley, G. T., & Mukherjee, P. (2008). Focal lesions in acute mild traumatic brain injury and neurocognitive outcome: CT versus 3T MRI. *Journal of Neurotrauma, 25*(9), 1049–1056.

Lee, L. K. (2007). Controversies in the sequelae of pediatric mild traumatic brain injury. *Pediatric Emergency Care, 23*(8), 580–586.

Lehr, E. (1990). *Psychological management of traumatic brain injuries in children and adolescents.* Rockville, MD: Aspen.

Leon-Carrion, J., & Ramos, F. J. (2003). Blows to the head during development can predispose to violent criminal behaviour: Rehabilitation of consequences of head injury is a measure for crime prevention. *Brain Injury, 17*(3), 207–216.

Leon-Carrion, J., Dominguez-Roldan, J. M., Leon-Dominguez, U., & Murillo-Cabezas, F. (2010). The infrascanner, a handheld device for screening in situ for the presence of brain haematomas. *Brain Injury, 24*(10), 1193–1201.

Lequerica, A. H., Rapport, L. L., Loeher, K., Axelrod, B. N., Vangel, S. J., & Hanks, R. A. (2007). Agitation in acquired brain injury: Impact on acute rehabilitation therapies. *Journal of Head Trauma Rehabilitation, 22*, 177–183.

Lescohier, I., & DiScala, C. (1993). Blunt trauma in children: Causes and outcomes of head versus intracranial injury. *Pediatrics, 91*, 721–725.

Levin, H. S., Amparco, E., Eisenberg, H. M., Williams, D., High, W., McArdle, C., . . . Weiner, R. L. (1987). Magnetic resonance imaging and computerised tomography in relation to the neurobehavioral sequelae of mild and moderate head injuries. *Journal of Neurosurgery, 66*, 706–713.

Levin, H. S., & Eisenberg, H. M. (1979). Neuropsychological impairment after closed head injury in children and adolescents. *Journal of Pediatric Psychology, 4*(4), 389–402.

Levin, H., Eisenberg, H. M., Wigg, N. R., & Kobayashi, K. (1982). Memory and intellectual ability after head injury in children and adolescents. *Neurosurgery, 11*, 668–673.

Levin, H. S., Grafman, J., & Eisenberg, H. M. (1987). *Neurobehavioral recovery from head injury.* New York, NY: Oxford University Press.

Levin, H. S., Hanten, G., & Li, X. (2009). The relation of cognitive control to social outcome after paediatric TBI: Implications for intervention. *Developmental Neurorehabilitation, 12*(5), 320–329.

Levin, H., Hanten, G., Max, J., Li, X., Swank, P., Ewing-Cobbs, L., . . . Schachar, R. (2007). Symptoms of attention-deficit/hyperactivity disorder following traumatic brain injury in children. *Journal of Developmental and Behavioral Pediatrics, 28*(2), 108–118.

Levin, H. S., Hanten, G., Roberson, G., Li, X., Ewing-Cobbs, L., Dennis, M., . . . Swank, P. (2008). Prediction of cognitive sequelae based on abnormal computed tomography findings in children following mild traumatic brain injury. *Journal of Neurosurgery Pediatrics, 1*(6), 461–470.

Levin, H. S., Hanten, G., Zhang, L., Swank, P. R., Ewing-Cobbs, L., Dennis, M., Barnes, M. A., Max, J., Schachar, R., Chapman, S. B., . . . Hunter, J. V. (2004). Changes in working memory after traumatic brain injury in children. *Neuropsychology, 18*(2), 240–247.

Levin, H. S., Hanten, G., Zhang, L., Swank, P. R., & Hunter, J. (2004). Selective impairment of inhibition after TBI in children. *Journal of Clinical and Experimental Neuropsychology, 26*(5), 589–597.

Levin, H., High, W., Ewing-Cobbs, L., Fletcher, J., Eisenberg, H. M., Miner, M. E., & Goldstein, F. C. (1988). Memory functioning during the first year after closed head injury in children and adolescents. *Neurosurgery, 22*(6), 1043–1052.

Levin, H., & Kraus, M. F. (1994). The frontal lobes and traumatic brain injury. *Journal of Neuropsychiatry and Clinical Neurosciences, 6*, 443–454.

Levin, H. S., Song, J., Ewing-Cobbs, L., & Roberson, G. (2001). Porteus Maze performance following traumatic brain injury in children. *Neuropsychology, 15*(4), 557–567.

Levin, H. S., Song, J., Scheibel, R. S., Fletcher, J. M., Harward, H., Lilly, M. M., & Goldstein, F. (1997). Concept formation and problem-solving following closed head injury in children. *Journal of the International Neuropsychological Society, 3*, 598–607.

Levin, H. S., Wilde, E. A., Chu, Z., Yallampalli, R., Hanten, G. R., Li, X., . . . Hunter, J. V. (2008). Diffusion tensor imaging in relation to cognitive and functional outcome of traumatic brain injury in children. *J Head Trauma Rehabil, 23*(4), 197–208.

Levin, H. S., Wilde, E., Troyanskaya, M., Petersen, N. J., Scheibel, R., Newsome, M., . . . Li, X. (2010). Diffusion tensor imaging of mild to moderate blast-related brain injury and its sequelae. *Journal of Neurotrauma, 27*, 583–594.

Levy, M., Berson, A., Cook, T., Bollegala, N., Seto, E., Tursanski, S., . . . Bhalerao, S. (2005). Treatment of agitation following traumatic brain injury: A review of the literature. *Neurorehabilitation, 20*, 279–306.

Lewine, J. D., Davis, J. T., Sloan, J. H., Kodituwakku, P. W., & Orrison, W. W., Jr. (1999). Neuromagnetic assessment of pathophysiologic brain activity induced by minor head trauma. *American Journal of Neuroradiology, 20*(5), 857–866.

Lezak, M. (1993). *Neuropsychological Assessment.* New York, Oxford University Press.

Lezak, M. (1995). *Neuropsychological assessment* (3rd ed.). New York, NY: Oxford.

Lezak, M. D., Howieson, D. B., & Loring, D. W. (2004). *Neuropsychological assessment* (4th ed.). New York, NY: Oxford University Press.

Li, L., & Liu, J. (2012). The effect of pediatric traumatic brain injury on behavioral outcomes: A systematic review. *Developmental Medicine & Child Neurology, 55*(1), 37–45.

Limond, J., Dorris, L., & McMillan, T. M. (2009). Quality of life in children with acquired brain injury: Parent perspectives 1–5 years after injury. *Brain Injury, 23*, 617–622.

Limond, J., & Leeke, R. (2005). Cognitive rehabilitation for children with acquired brain injury. *Journal of Child Psychology and Psychiatry, 46*(4), 339–352.

Linder-Lucht, M., Verena Othmer, D., Walther, M., Vry, J., Michaelis, U., Stein, S., . . . Mall, V. (2007). Validation of the Gross Motor Function Measure for use in children and adolescents with traumatic brain injuries. *Pediatrics, 120*(4), 880–886.

Lisa M. Moran, H. Gerry Taylor, Kalaichelvi Ganesalingam, Julie M. Gastier-Foster, Jessica Frick, Barbara Bangert, Ann Dietrich, Kathryn E. Nuss, Jerome Rusin, Martha Wright, and Keith O. Yeates. Apolipoprotein E4 as a Predictor of Outcomes in Pediatric Mild

Traumatic Brain Injury. *J Neurotrauma.* 2009 Sep; 26(9): 1489–1495. doi: 10.1089/neu. 2008.0767.PMCID: PMC2822810.

Ljungqvist, J., Nilsson, D., Ljungberg, M., Sorbo, A., Esbjornsson, E., Eriksson-Ritzen, C., . . . Skoglund, T. (2011). Longitudinal study of the diffusion tensor imaging properties of the corpus callosum in acute and chronic diffuse axonal injury. *Brain Injury, 25*(4), 370–378.

Lovell, M. R., & Collins, M. W. (1998). Neuropsychological assessment of the college football player. *Journal of Head Trauma Rehabilitation, 13(2),* 9–26.

Lovell, M. R., Collins, M. W., Iverson, G. L., Field, M., Maroon, J. C., Cantu, R. . . . Fu, F. H. (2003). Recovery from mild concussion in high school athletes. *Journal of Neurosurgery, 98(2),* 296–301.

Lovell, M. R., Collins, M. W., Podell, K., Powell, J., & Maroon, J. C. (2000). *ImPACT: Immediate post-concussion assessment and cognitive testing.* Pittsburgh, PA: NeuroHealth Systems, LLC.

Lowther, J. L., & Mayfield, J. (2004). Memory functioning in children with traumatic brain injuries: A TOMAL validity study. *Archives of Clinical Neuropsychology, 19,* 105–118.

Lumba, A. K., Schnadower, D., & Joseph, M. M. (2011). Evidence-based management of pediatric mild traumatic brain injury. *Pediatric Emergency Medicine Practice, 8,* 1–20.

Luton, L. M., Reed-Knight, B., Loiselle, K., O'Toole, K., & Blount, R. (2011). A pilot study evaluating an abbreviated version of the cognitive remediation programme for youth with neurocognitive deficits. *Brain Injury, 25*(4), 409–415.

Maas, A. I., & Menon, D. K. (2012). Traumatic brain injury: Rethinking ideas and approaches. *Lancet Neurology, 11,* 12–13.

Maas, A. I., Menon, D. K., Lingsma, H. F., Pineda, J. A., Sandel, M. E., & Manley, G. T. (2012). Re-orientation of clinical research in traumatic brain injury: Report of an international workshop on comparative effectiveness research. *Journal of Neurotrauma, 29,* 32–46.

MacKenzie, J., Siddiqi, F., Babb, J., Bagley, L., Mannon, L., Sinson, G., & Grossman, R. (2002). Brain atrophy in mild or moderate traumatic brain injury: A longitudinal quantitative analysis. *American Journal of Neuroradiology, 23*(9), 1509–1515.

Madsen-Sjo, N., Spellerberg, S., Weidner, S., & Kihlgren, M. (2010). Training of attention and memory deficits in children with acquired brain injury. *Acta Paediatrica, 99,* 230–236.

Maguire, S., Pickerd, N., Farewell, D., Mann, M., Tempest, V., & Kemp, A. M. (2009). Which clinical features distinguish inflicted from non-inflicted brain injury? A systematic review. *Archives of Disease in Childhood, 94*(11), 860–867.

Mahalick, D. M., Carmel, P. W., Greenberg, J. P., Molofsky, W., Brown, J. A., Heary, R. F., . . . von der Schmidt, E. III. (1998). Psychopharmacologic treatment of acquired attention disorders in children with brain injury. *Pediatric Neurosurgery, 29,* 121–126.

Maillard-Wermelinger, A., Yeates, K. O., Taylor, H. G., Rusin, J., Bangert, B., Dietrich, A., . . . Wright, M. (2009). Mild traumatic brain injury and executive functions in school-aged children. *Developmental Neurorehabilitation, 12*(5), 330–341.

Malec, J. F. (2009). Ethical and evidence-based practice in brain injury rehabilitation. *Neuropsychological Rehabilitation, 19*(6), 790–806.

Mandalis, A., Kinsella, G., Ong, B., & Anderson, V. (2007). Working memory and new learning following pediatric traumatic brain injury. *Developmental Neuropsychology, 32*(2), 683–701.

Mangeot, S., Armstrong, K., Colvin, A. N., Yeates, K. O., & Taylor, H. G. (2002). Long-term executive function deficits in children with traumatic brain injuries: Assessment using the Behavior Rating Inventory of Executive Function. *Child Neuropsychology, 8*(4), 271–284.

Manly, T., Anderson, V., Robertson, I., & Nimmo-Smith, I. (1999). *The Test of Everyday Attention for Children*. London: Thames Valley Test Company.

Manly, T., Robertson, R., Anderson V., & Crawford C. (in press). *The Test of Everyday Attention for Children* (2nd ed.). London: Pearson Publishers.

Marosszeky, N.E.V., Batchelor, J., Shores, E. A., Marosszeky, J. E., Klein-boonschate, M., & Fahey, P. P. (1993). The performance of hospitalized, non head-injured children on the Westmead PTA Scale. *Clinical Neuropsychologist, 7*(1), 85–95.

Marquardt, T. P., Stoll, J., & Sussman, H. (1988). Disorders of communication in acquired cerebral trauma. *Journal of Learning Disabilities, 21*(6), 340–351.

Marquez de la Plata, C. D., Garces, J., Shokri Kojori, E., Grinnan, J., Krishnan, K., Pidikiti, R., . . . Diaz-Arrastia, R. (2011). Deficits in functional connectivity of hippocampal and frontal lobe circuits after traumatic axonal injury. *Archives of Neurology, 68*(1), 74–84.

Marshall, S., Teasell, R., Bayona, N., Lippert, C., Chundamala, J., Villamere, J., . . . Bayley, M. (2007). Motor impairment rehabilitation post acquired brain injury. *Brain Injury, 21*(2), 133–160.

Masel, B. E., & DeWitt, D. S. (2010). Traumatic brain injury: A disease process, not an event. *Journal of Neurotrauma, 27*, 1529–1540.

Massagli, T. L., Fann, J. R., Burington, B. E., Jaffe, K. M., Katon, W. J., & Thompson, R. S. (2004). Psychiatric illness after mild traumatic brain injury in children. *Archives of Physical Medicine and Rehabilitation, 85*, 428–434.

Mateer, C. (1999). Executive function disorders: Rehabilitation challenges and strategies. *Seminars in Clinical Neuropsychiatry, 4*, 50–59.

Mateer, C., Kerns, K., & Eso, K. (2006). Management of attention and memory disorders following traumatic brain injury. *J Learning Disabilities, 29*, 6118–6132.

Mateer, C. A., & Sira, C. S. (2006). Cognitive and emotional consequences of TBI: Intervention strategies for vocational rehabilitation. *NeuroRehabilitation, 21*(4), 315–326.

Matsukawa, H., Shinoda, M., Fujii, M., Takahashi, O., Murakata, A., Yamamoto, D., . . . Ishikawa, R. (2011). Intraventricular hemorrhage on computed tomography and corpus callosum injury on magnetic resonance imaging in patients with isolated blunt traumatic brain injury. *Journal of Neurosurgery, 117*, 334–339.

Max, J. E., Kaetley, E., Wilde, E. A., Bigler, E. D., Schachar, R. J., Saunders, A., . . . Yang, T. T. (2011). Anxiety disorders in children and adolescents in the first six months after traumatic brain injury. *Journal of Neuropsychiatry and Clinical Neurosciences, 23*(1), 29–39.

Max, J., Lindgren, S., Knutson, C., Pearson, S., Ihrig, D., & Welborn, A. (1998). Child and adolescent traumatic brain injury: Correlates of disruptive behavior disorders. *Brain Injury, 12*, 41–52.

Mayer, A. R., Ling, J. M., Yang, Z., Pena, A., Yeo, R. A., & Klimaj, S. (2012). Diffusion abnormalities in pediatric mild traumatic brain injury. *Neurobiology of Disease, 32*(50), 17961–17969.

Mayer, A. R., Mannell, M.V., Ling, J., Gasparovic, C., & Yeo, R. A. (2011). Functional connectivity in mild traumatic brain injury. *Human Brain Mapping, 32*(11), 1825–1835.

Mazaux, J. M., & Richer, E. (1998). Rehabilitation after traumatic brain injury in adults. *Disability and Rehabilitation, 21*, 435–447.

McCauley, S. R., & Levin, H. S. (2004). Prospective memory in pediatric traumatic brain injury: A preliminary study. *Developmental Neuropsychology, 25*(1&2), 5–20.

McCauley, S. R., Wilde, E. A., Bigler, E. D., Chu, Z., Yallampalli, R., Oni, M. B., . . . Levin, H. S. (2011). Diffusion tensor imaging of incentive effects in prospective memory after pediatric traumatic brain injury. *Journal of Neurotrauma, 28*(4), 503–516.

McCrea, M. (2001a). Standardized mental status assessment of sports concussion. *Clinical Journal of Sport Medicine, 11*, 176–181.

McCrea, M. (2001b). Standardized mental status testing on the sideline after sport-related concussion. *Journal of Athletic Training, 36*(3), 274–279.

McCrea, M., Kelly, J. P., Kluge, J., Ackley, B., & Randolph, C. (1997). Standardized assessment of concussion in football players. *Neurology, 48,* 586–588.

McCrea, M., Kelly, J. P., & Randolph, C. (2000). *Standardized assessment of concussion (SAC): Manual for administration, scoring and interpretation* (3rd ed.). Waukesha, WI: Comprehensive Neuropsychological Services.

McCrea, M., Kelly, J. P., Randolph, C., Kluge, J., Bartolic, E., Ginn, G., & Baxter, B. (1998). Standardized assessment of concussion (SAC): On-site mental status evaluation of the athlete. *Journal of Head Trauma Rehabilitation, 13,* 27–35.

McCrory, P. (2011). Future advances and areas of future focus in the treatment of sport-related concussion. *Clinical Sports Medicine, 30,* 201–208.

McCrory, P., Collie, A., & Anderson, V. (2004). Can we manage sport-related concussion in children the same as in adults? *British Journal of Sports Medicine, 38,* 516–519.

McCrory, P., Johnston, K., Meeuwisse, W., Aubry, M., Cantu, R., Dvorak, J., . . . Schamasch, P. (2005). Summary and agreement statement of the 2nd international conference on concussion in sport, Prague 2004. *British Journal of Sports Medicine, 39,* 196–204.

McCrory, P., Meeuwisse, W., Aubry, M., Cantu, B., Dvorak, J., & Echemendia, R. (2013). Consensus statement on concussion in sport: The 4th International Conference on Concussion in Sport, held in Zurich. *British Journal of Sports Medicine, 47,* 250–258.

McCrory, P., Meeuwisse, W., Johnston, K., Dvorak, J., Aubry, M., Molloy, M., & Cantu, R. (2009). Consensus Statement on Concussion in Sport: The 3rd International Conference on Concussion in Sport Held in Zurich, November 2008. *The Physician and Sportsmedicine, 37*(2), 141–159.

McDonald, B. C., Saykin, A. J., & McAllister, T. W. (2012). Functional MRI of mild and traumatic brain injury (mTBI): Progress and perspectives from the first decade. *Brain Imaging and Behavior, 6,* 193–207.

McDowell, S., Whyte, J., & D'Esposito, M. (1997). Working memory impairments in traumatic brain injury: Evidence from a dual-task paradigm. *Neuropsychologica, 35,* 1341–1353.

McKay, C. D., Brooks, B. L., Mrazik, M., Jubinville, A. L., & Emery, C. A. (2014). Psychometric properties and reference values for the ImPACT neurocognitive test battery in a sample of elite youth ice hockey players. *Arch Clin Neuropsychol, 29*(2): 141–151.

McKay, K. E., Halperin, J. M., Schwartz, S. T., & Sharma, V. (1994). Developmental analysis of three aspects of information processing: Sustained attention, selective attention and response organisation. *Developmental Neuropsychology, 10*(2), 121–132.

McKinlay, A. (2009). Controversies and outcomes associated with mild traumatic brain injury in childhood and adolescences. *Child: Care, Health and Development, 36*(1), 3–21.

McKinlay, A., Dalrymple-Alford, J. C., Horwood, L. J., & Fergusson, D. M. (2002). Long term psychosocial outcomes after mild head injury in early childhood. *Journal of Neurology, Neurosurgery, and Psychiatry, 73,* 281–288.

McKinlay, A., Grace, R., Horwood, L, & Fergusson, D. (2008). Prevalence of traumatic brain injury among children, adolescents and young adults: Prospective evidence from a birth cohort. *Brain Injury, 22,* 175–181.

McKinlay, A., Grace, R. C., Horwood, L. J., Fergusson, D. M., & MacFarlane, M. R. (2009). Long-term behavioural outcomes of pre-school mild traumatic brain injury. *Child: Care, Health and Development, 36*(1), 22–30.

McKinlay, A., Kyonka, E.G.E., Grace, R. C., Horwood, L. J., Fergusson, D. M., & MacFarlane, M. R. (2010). An investigation of the pre-injury risk factors associated with children who experience brain injury. *Injury Prevention, 16,* 31–35.

McLean, D. E., Kaitz, E. S., Kennan, C. J., Dabney, K., Cawley, M. F., & Alexander, M. A. (1995). Medical and surgical complications of pediatric brain injury. *Journal of Head Trauma Rehabilitation, 10*, 1–12.

Merkley, T. L., Bigler, E. D., Wilde, E. A., McCauley, S. R., Hunter, J. V., & Levin, H. S. (2008). Diffuse changes in cortical thickness in pediatric moderate-to-severe traumatic brain injury. *Journal of Neurotrauma, 25*(11), 1343–1345.

Michaud, L. J., Rivara, F. P., Grady, M. S., & Reay, D. T. (1992). Predictors of survival and severe disability after severe brain injury in children. *Neurosurgery, 31*, 254–264.

Miles, L., Grossman, R. I., Johnson, G., Babb, J. S., Diller, L., & Inglese, M. (2008). Short-term DTI predictors of cognitive dysfunction in mild traumatic brain injury. *Brain Injury, 22*(2), 115–122.

Miller, J. D. (1991). Pathophysiology and management of head injury. *Neuropsychology, 5*, 235–261.

Miller, L. (1996). Neuropsychology and pathophysiology of mild head injury and the post-concussion syndrome: Clinical and forensic considerations. *The Journal of Cognitive Rehabilitation, 15*, 8–23.

Mirsky, A. F., Anthony, B. J., Duncan, C. C., Ahearn, M. B., & Kellam, S. G. (1991). Analysis of the elements of attention: A neuropsychological approach. *Neuropsychology Review, 2*(2), 109–145.

Moran, L. M., Taylor, H. G., Rusin, J., Bangert, B., Dietrich, A., Nuss, K. E., . . . Yeates, K. O. (2012). Quality of life in pediatric mild traumatic brain injury and its relationship to postconcussive symptoms. *Journal of Pediatric Psychology, 37*(7), 736–744.

Morris, K. P., Forsyth, R. J., Parslow, R. C., Tasker, R. C., & Hawley, C. A. (2006). Intracranial pressure complicating severe traumatic brain injury in children: Monitoring and management. *Intensive Care Medicine, 32*, 1606–1612.

Morse, S., Haritou, F., Ong, B., Anderson, V., Catroppa, C., & Rosenfeld, J. (1999). Early effect of traumatic brain injury on young children's language performance: A preliminary linguistic analysis. *Pediatric Rehabilitation, 3*(4), 139–148.

Mottram, L., & Berger-Gross, P. (2004). An intervention to reduce disruptive behaviours in children with brain injury. *Pediatric Rehabilitation, 7*(2), 133–143.

Msall, M. E., DiGaudio, K., Rogers, B. T., LaForest, S., Catanzaro, N. L., Campbell, J. . . . Duffy, L. C. (1994). The Functional Independence Measure for Children (WeeFIM). Conceptual basis and pilot use in children with developmental disabilities. *Clinical Pediatrics, 33*(7), 421–430.

Muller, R. A., Behen, M. E., Rothermel, R. D., Muzik, O., Chakraborty, P. K., & Chugani, H. T. (1999). Brain organization for language in children, adolescents, and adults with left hemisphere lesion: A PET study. *Progress in Neuro-Psychopharmacology and Biological Psychiatry, 23*(4), 657–668.

Munson, S., Schroth, E., & Ernst, M. (2006). The role of functional neuroimaging in pediatric brain injury. *Pediatrics, 117*(4), 1372–1381.

Muscara, F., Catroppa, C., & Anderson, V. (2008a). The impact of injury severity on executive function 7–10 years following pediatric traumatic brain injury. *Developmental Neuropsychology, 5*, 623–636.

Muscara, F., Catroppa, C., & Anderson, V. (2008b). Social problem-solving skills as a mediator between executive function and long-term social outcome following paediatric traumatic brain injury. *Journal of Neuropsychology, 2*(2), 445–461.

Muscara, F., & Crowe, L. (2012). Measuring social skills with questionnaires and rating scales. In V. Anderson & M. H. Beauchamp (Eds.), *Developmental social neuroscience and childhood brain insult: Theory and practice* (pp. 119–137). New York, NY: Guilford Press.

Mysiw, W. J., & Sandel, M. E. (1997). The agitated brain injured patient: Part 2: Pathophysiology and treatment. *Archives of Physical and Medical Rehabilitation, 78*, 213–220.

Nadebaum, C., Anderson, V., & Catroppa, C. (2007). Executive function outcomes following traumatic brain injury in young children: A five year follow-up. *Developmental Neuropsychology, 32*(2), 703–728.

Napolitano, E., Elovic, E. P., & Qureshi, A. I. (2005). Pharmacological stimulant treatment of neurocognitive and functional deficits after traumatic and non-traumatic brain injury. *Medical Science Monitor, 11*(6), 212–220.

National Collaborating Centre for Acute Care. (2007). *Head injury: Triage, assessment, investigation, and early management of head injury in infants, children and adults.* London: National Institute for Health and Clinical Excellence.

National Pediatric Trauma Registry. (1993). *Summary of findings.* Boston, MA: Research and Training Center on Childhood Trauma.

Newsome, M. R., Scheibel, R. S., Hunter, J. V., Wang, Z. J., Chu, Z., Li, X., . . . Levin, H. S. (2007). Brain activation during working memory after traumatic brain injury in children. *Neurocase, 13*(1), 16–24.

Newsome, M. R., Scheibel, R. S., Steinberg, J. L., Troyanskaya, M., Sharma, R. G., Rauch, R. A., . . . Levin, H. S. (2007). Working memory brain activation following severe traumatic brain injury. *Cortex, 43*(1), 95–111.

Niedzwecki, C. M., Marwitz, J. H., Ketchum, J. M., Cifu, D. X., Dillard, C. M., & Monasterio, E. A. (2008). Traumatic brain injury: A comparison of inpatient functional outcomes between children and adults. *Journal of Head Trauma Rehabilitation, 23*(4), 209–219.

NINDS Common Data Elements. (2015). Traumatic brain injury. Retrieved from http://www.commondataelements.ninds.nih.gov/TBI.aspx

Noggle, C. A., & Pierson, E. E. (2010). Psychosocial and behavioral functioning following pediatric TBI: Presentation, assessment, and intervention. *Applied Neuropsychology, 17*, 110–115.

North, B. (1984). *Jamieson's first notebook of head injury* (3rd ed.). London: Butterworths.

Norup, A., Siert, L., & Lykke Mortensen, E. (2010). Emotional distress and quality of life in relatives of patients with severe brain injury: The first month after injury. *Brain Injury, 24*(2), 81–88.

Novack, T. A., Dillon, M. C., & Jackson, W. T. (1996). Neurochemical mechanisms in brain injury and treatment: A review. *Journal of Clinical and Experimental Neuropsychology, 18*, 685–706.

Nucleus Medical Media. (2015). Axon Shear (Post-concussion Syndrome). *Nucleus Catalog.* Retrieved July 7, 2015, from http://www.nucleuscatalog.com/axon-shear-post-concussion-syndrome/view-item?ItemID=1870

Nybo, T., & Koskiniemi, M. (1999). Cognitive indicators of vocational outcome after severe traumatic brain injury in childhood. *Brain Injury, 13*(10), 759–766.

Nybo, T., Sainio, M., & Muller, K. (2004). Stability of vocational outcome in adulthood after moderate to severe preschool brain injury. *Journal of the International Neuropsychological Society, 10*(5), 719–723.

Oberg, L., & Turkstra, L. (1998). Use of elaborative encoding to facilitate verbal learning after adolescent traumatic brain injury. *Journal of Head Trauma Rehabilitation, 13*, 44–62.

Olsson, K. A., Lloyd, O. T., Lebrocque, R. M., Mckinlay, L., Anderson, V. A., & Kenardy, J. A. (2013). Predictors of child post-concussion symptoms at 6 and 18 months following mild traumatic brain injury. *Brain Injury, 27*(2), 145–157.

Ommaya, A., Goldsmith, W., & Thibault, L. (2002). Biomechanics and neuropathology of adult and pediatric head injury. *British Journal of Neurosurgery, 16*, 220–242.

O'Neill, J. H., Zuger, R. R., Fields, A., Fraser, R., & Pruce, T. (2004). The Program Without Walls: Innovative approach to state agency rehabilitation of persons with traumatic brain injury. *Archives of Physical and Medical Rehabilitation, 85*(2), S68–S72.

Ornstein, T. J., Levin, H. S., Chen, S., Hanten, G., Ewing-Cobbs, L., Dennis, M., . . . Schachar, R. (2009). Performance monitoring in children following traumatic brain injury. *Journal of Child Psychology and Psychiatry and Allied Disciplines, 50*(4), 506–513.

Osmond, M. H., Klassen, T. P., Wells, G. A., Correll, R., Jarvis, A., Joubert, G., . . . Stiell, I. G. (2010). CATCH: A clinical decision rule for the use of computed tomography in children with minor head injury. *Canadian Medical Association Journal, 182*(4), 341–348.

Ostberg, A., Virta, J., Rinne, J. O., Oikonen, V., Luoto, P., Nagren, K., . . . Tenovuo, O. (2011). Cholinergic dysfunction after traumatic brain injury: Preliminary findings from a PET study. *Neurology, 76*(12), 1046–1050.

Owens, J. A., Spirito, A., & McGuinn, M. (2000). The Children's Sleep Habits Questionnaire (CSHQ): Psychometric properties of a survey instrument for school-aged children. *Sleep (New York), 23*, 1043–1052.

Ownsworth, T., & McKenna, K. (2004). Investigation of factors related to employment outcome following traumatic brain injury: A critical review and conceptual model. *Disability and Rehabilitation, 26*(13), 765–783.

Pang, D. (1985). Pathophysiologic correlates of neurobehavioral syndromes following closed head injury. In M. Ylvisaker (Ed.), *Head injury rehabilitation: Children and adolescents* (pp. 3–70). London: Taylor & Francis.

Papero, P., Prigatano, G., Snyder, H., & Johnson, D. (1993). Children's adaptive behavioral competence after head injury. *Neuropsychological Rehabilitation, 3*(4), 321–340.

Pardes Berger, R., Beers, S. R., Rochichi, R., Wiesman, D., & Adelson, P. D. (2007). Serum biomarker concentrations and outcome after pediatric traumatic brain injury. *Journal of Neurotrauma, 24*, 1793–1801.

Park, B., Allen, D., Barney, S., Ringdahl, E., & Mayfield, J. (2009). Structure of attention in children with traumatic brain injury. *Applied Neuropsychology, 16*, 1–10.

Park, N., & Ingles, J. (2001). Effectiveness of attention rehabilitation after acquired brain injury: A meta-analysis. *Neuropsychology, 15*, 199–210.

Parker, J. G., & Asher, S. R. (1989). Friendship Quality Questionnaire—Revised: Instructions and Manual. University of Michigan.

Parker, J., & Asher, S. (1993). Friendship and friendship quality in middle childhood: Links with peer group acceptance and feelings of loneliness and social dissatisfaction. *Developmental Psychology, 29*(4), 611–621.

Parslow, R. C., Morris, K. P., Tasker, R. C., Forsyth, R. J., & Hawley, C. A. (2005). Epidemiology of traumatic brain injury in children receiving intensive care in the UK. *Archives of Disease in Childhood, 90*, 1182–1187.

Penkman, L. (2004). Remediation of attention deficits in children: A focus on childhood cancer, traumatic brain injury and attention deficit disorder. *Pediatric Rehabilitation, 7*(2), 111–123.

Penn, P. R., Rose, F. D., & Johnson, D. A. (2009). Virtual enriched environments in paediatric neuropsychological rehabilitation following traumatic brain injury: Feasibility, benefits and challenges. *Developmental Neurorehabilitation, 12*(1), 32–43.

Pentland, L., Todd, J. A., & Anderson, V. (1998). The impact of head injury severity on planning ability in adolescence: A functional analysis. *Neuropsychological Rehabilitation, 8*, 301–317.

Perdices, M., & Tate, R. L. (2009). Single-subject designs as a tool for evidence-based clinical practice: Are they unrecognised and undervalued? *Neuropsychological Rehabilitation, 19*(6), 904–927.

Peterson, R. L., Kirkwood, M. W., Taylor, H. G., Stancin, T., Brown, T. M., & Wade, S. L. (2013). Adolescents' internalizing problems following traumatic brain injury are related to parents' psychiatric symptoms. *J Head Trauma Rehabil, 28*(5): E1–E12.

Pettit, G. S., Dodge, K. A., & Brown, M. M. (1988). Early family experience, social problem solving patterns, and children's social competence. *Child Development, 59*, 107–120.

Philip, S., Udomphorn, Y., Kirkham, F. J., & Vavilala, M. S. (2009). Cerebrovascular pathophysiology in pediatric traumatic brain injury. *The Journal of Trauma, Injury, Infection, and Critical Care, 67*(2 Suppl.), S128–134.

Piazza, O., Storti, M. P., Cotena, S., Stoppa, F., Perrotta, D., Esposito, G., . . . Tufano, R. (2007). S100B is not a reliable prognostic index in paediatric TBI. *Pediatric Neurosurgery, 43*(4), 258–264.

Pinto, P. S., Meoded, A., Poretti, A., Tekes, A., & Huisman, T. A. (2012). The unique features of traumatic brain injury in children. Review of the characteristics of the pediatric skull and brain, mechanisms of trauma, patterns of injury, complications, and their imaging findings—part 2. *J Neuroimaging, 22*(2), e18–e41.

Pinto, P. S., Poretti, A., Meoded, A., Tekes, A., & Huisman, T. A. (2012). The unique features of traumatic brain injury in children. Review of the characteristics of the pediatric skull and brain, mechanisms of trauma, patterns of injury, complications, and their imaging findings—part 1. *J Neuroimaging, 22*(2), e1–e17.

Pinto PS1, Poretti A, Meoded A, Tekes A, Huisman TA. The unique features of traumatic brain injury in children. Review of the characteristics of the pediatric skull and brain, mechanisms of trauma, patterns of injury, complications and their imaging findings—part 1. *J Neuroimaging.* 2012 Apr; 22(2):e1-e17. doi: 10.1111/j.1552-6569.2011.00688.x. Epub 2012 Jan 24.

Pinto PS1, Meoded A, Poretti A, Tekes A, Huisman TA. The unique features of traumatic brain injury in children. Review of the characteristics of the pediatric skull and brain, mechanisms of trauma, patterns of injury, complications, and their imaging findings—part 2. *J Neuroimaging.* 2012 Apr; 22(2):e18-41. doi: 10.1111/j.1552-6569.2011.00690.x. Epub 2012 Feb 3.

Poggi, G., Liscio, M., Adduci, A., Galbiatti, S., Massimino, M., Sommovigo, M., . . . Castelli, E. (2005). Psychological and adjustment problems due to acquired brain lesions in childhood: A comparison between post-traumatic patients and brain tumour survivors. *Brain Injury, 19*(10), 777–785.

Polderman, K. H. (2009). Mechanisms of action, physiological effects, and complications of hypothermia. *Critical Care and Medicine, 37*, 186–202.

Ponsford, J., Draper, K., & Schonberger, M. (2008). Functional outcome 10 years after traumatic brain injury: Its relationship with demographic, injury severity, and cognitive and emotional status. *Journal of the International Neuropsychological Society, 14*(2), 233–242.

Ponsford, J., Sloan, S., & Snow, P. (1995). *Traumatic brain injury: Rehabilitation for everyday adaptive living.* Hove, UK: Lawrence Erlbaum Associates.

Ponsford, J., Willmott, C., Rothwell, A., Cameron, P., Ayton, G., Nelms, R., . . . Ng, K. T. (1999). Cognitive and behavioural outcomes following mild traumatic head injury in children. *Journal of Head Trauma Rehabilitation, 14*, 360–372.

Ponsford, J., Willmott, C., Rothwell, A., Cameron, P., Ayton, G., Nelms, R., . . . Ng, K. (2001). Impact of early intervention on outcome after mild traumatic brain injury in children. *Pediatrics, 108*(6), 1297–1303.

Posner, M. I., & Peterson, S. E. (1990). The attention system of the human brain. *Annual Review of Neuroscience, 13*, 25–42.

Povlishock, J. T. (1993). Pathobiology of traumatically induced axonal injury in animals and man. *Annals of Emergency Medicine, 22*(6), 980–986.

Povlishock, J. T., & Katz, D. I. (2005). Update of neuropathology and neurological recovery after traumatic brain injury. *Journal of Head Trauma Rehabilitation, 20*, 76–94.

Powell, J. M., Temkin, N. R., Machamer, J. E., & Dikmen, S. S. (2002). Nonrandomized studies of rehabilitation for traumatic brain injury: Can they determine effectiveness? *Archives of Physical Medicine and Rehabilitation, 83*, 1235–1244.

Prange, M., & Margulies, S. (2002). Regional, directional, and age-dependent properties of brain undergoing large deformation. *Journal of Biomechanical Engineering, 124*, 244–252.

Pressdee, D., May, L., Eastman, E., & Grier, D. (1997). The use of play therapy in the preparation of children undergoing MR imaging. *Clinical Radiology, 52*(12), 945–947.

Prigatano, G. P., & Gray, J. A. (2007). Parental concerns and distress after paediatric traumatic brain injury: A qualitative study. *Brain Injury, 21*(7), 721–729.

Prigatano, G., & Gray, J. A. (2008). Predictors of performance on three developmentally sensitive neuropsychological tests in children with and without traumatic brain injury. *Brain Injury, 22*(6), 491–500.

Prigatano, G., & Gupta, S. (2006). Friends after traumatic brain injury in children. *Journal of Head Trauma Rehabilitation, 21*(6), 505–513.

Prins, M., Giza, C., & Hovda, D. (2010). Neurobiology of TBI sustained during development. In V. Anderson & K. O. Yeates (Eds.), *Pediatric traumatic brain injury* (pp. 18–35). Cambridge, UK: Cambridge University Press.

Provenzale, J. M. (2010). Imaging of traumatic brain injury: A review of the recent medical literature. *Neuroradiology/Head and Neck Imaging Review, 194*, 16–19.

Purcell, L. (2009). What are the most appropriate return-to-play guidelines for concussed child athletes? *British Journal of Sports Medicine, 43*, i51–i55.

Quattrocchi, K., Prasad, P., Willits, N., & Wagner, F. (1991). Quantification of midline shift as a predictor of poor outcome following head injury. *Surgical Neurology, 35*, 183–188.

Raghubar, K. P., Barnes, M. A., Prasad, M., Johnson, C. P., & Ewing-Cobbs, L. (2013). Mathematical outcomes and working memory in children with TBI and orthopedic injury. *Journal of the International Neuropsychological Society, 19*, 1–10.

Raimondi, A., & Hirschauer, J. (1984). Head injury in the infant and toddler. *Child's Brain, 11*, 12–35.

Rapee, R., Lyneham, H., Schniering, C., Wuthrish, V., Abbott, M., Hudson, J., & Wignall, A. (2006). *Cool Kids* (School version).

Rappaport, M., & Hall, K. M. (1982). Disability rating scale for severe head trauma: Coma to community. *Archives of Physical Medicine and Rehabilitation, 63*, 118–123.

Raschle, N. M., Lee, M., Buechler, R., Christodoulou, J. A., Chang, M., Vakil, M., . . . Gaab, N. (2009). Making MR imaging child's play—pediatric neuroimaging protocol, guidelines and procedure. *J Vis Exp*(29).

Raschle, N., Zuk, J., Ortiz-Mantilla, S., Sliva, D. D., Franceschi, A., Grant, P. E., . . . Gaab, N. (2012). Pediatric neuroimaging in early childhood and infancy: Challenges and practical guidelines. *Ann N Y Acad Sci, 1252*, 43–50.

Rebok, G. W., Smith, C. B., Pascualvaca, D. M., Mirsky, A. F., Anthony, B. J., & Kellam, S. G. (1997). Developmental changes in attentional performance in urban children from eight to thirteen years. *Child Neuropsychology, 3*(1), 28–46.

Reilly, P. L., Simpson, D. A., Sprod, R., & Thomas, L. (1988). Assessing the conscious level in infants and young children: A paediatric version of the Glasgow Coma Scale. *Childs Nervous System, 4*(1), 30–33.

Reynolds, C. R., & Kamphaus, R. W. (1992). *Behavior assessment system for children*. Circle Pines, MN: American Guidance Service.

Rigotti, D. J., Inglese, M., & Gonen, O. (2007). Whole-brain n-acetylaspartate as a surrogate marker of neuronal damage in diffuse neurologic disorders. *American Journal of Neuroradiology, 28*(10), 1843–1849.

Rivara, F. P., Koepsell, T., Wang, J., Temkin, N., Dorsch, A., Vavilala, M. S., . . . Jaffe, K. M. (2011). Disability 3, 12, and 24 months after traumatic brain injury among children and adolescents. *Pediatrics, 128*(5), e1129–e1139.

Rivara, J. B., Jaffe, K. M., Fay, G. C., Polissar, N. L., Martin, K. M., Shurtleff, H. A., & Liao, S. (1993). Family functioning and injury severity as predictors of child functioning one year following traumatic brain injury. *Archives of Physical Medicine and Rehabilitation, 74*, 1047–1055.

Rivara, J., Jaffe, K., Polissar, N., Fay, G., Martin, K., Shurtleff, H., . . . Liao, S. (1994). Family functioning and children's academic performance in the year following traumatic brain injury. *Archives of Physical Medicine and Rehabilitation, 75*, 369–379.

Roberts, M., Manshad, F., Bushnell, D., & Hines, M. (1995). Neurobehavioral dysfunction following mild traumatic brain injury in childhood: A case report with positive findings on positron emission tomography (PET). *Brain Injury, 9*, 427–436.

Roberts, R. M., Mathias, J. L., & Rose, S. E. (2014). Diffusion Tensor Imaging (DTI) findings following pediatric non-penetrating TBI: A meta-analysis. *Dev Neuropsychol, 39*(8), 600–637.

Robertson, I. (1990). Does computerised cognitive rehabilitation work? A review. *Aphasiology, 4*, 381–405.

Robinson, K., Kaizar, E., Catroppa, C., Godfrey, C., & Yeates, K. O. (2014). Systematic review and meta-analysis of cognitive interventions for children with central nervous system disorders and neurodevelopmental disorders. *Journal of Pediatric Psychology, 39*(8), 846–865.

Rocca, A., Wallen, M., & Batchelor, J. (2008). The Westmead Post-Traumatic Amnesia Scale for Children (WPTAS-C) aged 4 and 5 years old. *Brain Impairment, 9*(1), 14–21.

Rosazza, C., & Minati, L. (2011). Resting-state brain networks: Literature review and clinical applications. *Neurol Sci, 32*(5), 773–785.

Rosema, S., Muscara, F., Anderson, V., Godfrey, C., Eren, S., & Catroppa, C. (2014). Young adults' perspectives on their psychosocial outcomes 16 years following childhood traumatic brain injury. *Social Care and Disability, 5*, 136–144.

Rosenberg, D. R., Sweeney, J. A., Gillen, J. S., Kim, J., Varanelli, M. J., O'Hearn, K. M., . . . et Thulborn, K. R. (1997). Magnetic resonance imaging of children without sedation: Preparation with simulation. *Journal of the American Academy of Child and Adolescent Psychiatry, 36*(6), 853–859.

Ross, D. E. (2011). Review of longitudinal studies of MRI brain volumetry in patients with traumatic brain injury. *Brain Injury, 25*(13–14), 1271–1278.

Ross, K. A., Dorris, L., & McMillan, T. (2011). A systematic review of psychological interventions to alleviate cognitive and psychosocial problems in children with acquired brain injury. *Developmental Medicine & Child Neurology, 53*(8), 692–701.

Rothi, L., & Horner, J. (1983). Restitution and substitution: Two theories of recovery with application to neurobehavioral treatment. *Journal of Clinical Neuropsychology, 3*, 73–81.

Rowley, G., & Fielding, K. (1991). Reliability and accuracy of the Glasgow Coma Scale with experienced and inexperienced users. *Lancet, 337*(8740), 535–538.

Ruijs, M. B., Keyser, A., & Gabreels, F. J. (1992). Assessment of post-traumatic amnesia in young children. *Dev Med Child Neurol, 34*(10), 885–892.

Runyan, D. K. (2008). The challenges of assessing the incidence of inflicted traumatic brain injury: A world perspective. *American Journal of Preventive Medicine, 34*(4 Suppl), S112–115.

Runyan, D. K., Berger, R. P., & Barr, R. G. (2008). Defining an ideal system to establish the incidence of inflicted traumatic brain injury: Summary of the consensus conference. *American Journal of Preventive Medicine, 34*(4 Suppl), S163–168.

Russo, R. N., Rice, J., Chern, P. M., & Raftos, J. (2012). Minimal and mild paediatric brain injury: A 3-year cohort of consecutive presentations. *Developmental Neurorehabilitation, 15*(1), 13–18.

Rutter, M., Chadwick, O., & Shaffer, D. (1983). Head injury. In M. Rutter (Ed.), *Developmental neuropsychiatry* (pp. 83–111). New York, NY: Guilford Press.

Ryan, N. P., Catroppa, C., Cooper, R. J., Beare, R., Ditchfield, M., Coleman, L., . . . Anderson, V. (2015). Relationships between acute imaging biomarkers and theory of mind impairment in post-acute pediatric traumatic brain injury: A prospective analysis using susceptibility weighted imaging (SWI). *Neuropsychologia, 66,* 32–38.

Sahuquillo, J., & Vilalta, A. (2007). Cooling the injured brain: Does moderate hypothermia influence the pathophysiology of traumatic brain injury? *Current Pharmaceutical Design, 13,* 2310–2322.

Salorio, C., Slomine, B., Grados, M. A., Vasa, R., Christensen, J., & Gerring, J. (2005). Neuroanatomic correlates of CVLT-C performance following pediatric traumatic brain injury. *Journal of the International Neuropsychological Society, 11,* 686–696.

Salorio, C. F., Slomine, B. S., Guerguerian, A., Christensen, J. R., White, J. R., Natale, J. E., . . . Gerring, J. P. (2008). Intensive care unit variables and outcome after pediatric traumatic brain injury: A retrospective study of survivors. *Pediatric Critical Care Medicine, 9*(1), 47–53.

Sander, A. M., Clark, A. N., & Pappadis, M. R. (2010). What is community integration anyway? Defining meaning following traumatic brain injury. *Journal of Head Trauma Rehabilitation, 25*(2), 121–127.

Sandler, S. J. I., Figaji, A. A., & Adelson, P. D. (2010). Clinical applications of biomarkers in pediatric traumatic brain injury. *Child's Nervous System, 26*(2), 205–213.

Sbordone, R. J. (2001). Limitations of neuropsychological testing to predict the cognitive and behavioral functioning of persons with brain injury in real-world settings. *NeuroRehabilitation, 16*(4), 199–201.

Scherwath, A., Sommerfeldt, D. W., Bindt, C., Nolte, A., Boiger, A., Koch, U., . . . Petersen-Ewert, C. (2011). Identifying children and adolescents with cognitive dysfunction following mild traumatic brain injury—Preliminary findings on abbreviated neuropsychological testing. *Brain Injury, 25*(4), 401–408.

Schmidt, A. T., Hanten, G., Li, X., Wilde, E. A., Ibarra, A. P., Chu, Z. D., . . . Levin, H. S. (2013). Emotional prosody and diffusion tensor imaging in children after traumatic brain injury. *Brain Injury, 27*(13–14), 1528–1535.

Schmidt, A. T., Hanten, G. R., Xiaodi, L., Vasquez, A. C., Wilde, E. A., Chapman, S. B., . . . Levin, H. S. (2012). Decision making after pediatric traumatic brain injury: Trajectory of recovery and relationship to age and gender. *International Journal of Developmental Neuroscience, 30,* 225–230.

Schmitter-Edgecombe, M., Fahy, J., Whelan, J., & Long, C. (1995). Memory remediation after severe head injury: Notebook training versus supportive therapy. *Journal of Consulting and Clinical Psychology, 63,* 484–489.

Schutzman, S., Barnes, P., Duhaime, A. C., Greenes, D., Homer, C., Jaffe, D., . . . Schunk, J. (2001). Evaluation and management of children younger than two years old with apparently minor head trauma: Proposed guidelines. *Pediatrics, 107*(5), 983–993.

Selznick, L., & Savage, R. C. (2000). Using self-monitoring procedures to increase on-task behavior with three adolescent boys with brain injury. *Behavioral Interventions, 15,* 243–260.

Semrud-Clikeman, M. (2010). Pediatric traumatic brain injury: Rehabilitation and transition to home and school. *Applied Neuropsychology, 17*, 116–122.

Senathi-Raja, D., Ponsford, J., & Schonberger, M. (2010). The association of age and time postinjury with long-term emotional outcome following traumatic brain injury. *Journal of Head Trauma Rehabilitation, 25*(5), 330–338.

Serra-Grabulosa, J. M., Junque, C., Verger, K., Salgado-Pineda, P., Maneru, C., & Mercader, J. M. (2005). Cerebral correlates of declarative memory dysfunctions in early traumatic brain injury. *J Neurol Neurosurg Psychiatry, 76*(1), 129–131.

Servadei, F., Compagnone, C., & Sahuquillo, J. (2007). The role of surgery in traumatic brain injury. *Current Opinion in Critical Care, 13*, 163–168.

Sesma, H., Slomine, B., Ding, R., & McCarthy, M. L. (2009). Executive functioning in the first year after pediatric traumatic brain injury. *Pediatrics, 121*(6), 1686–1695.

Shames, J., Treger, I., Ring, H., & Giaquinto, S. (2007). Return to work following traumatic brain injury: Trends and challenges. *Disability and Rehabilitation, 29*(17), 1387–1395.

Shenton, M. E., Hamoda, H. M., Schneiderman, S., Bouix, S., Pasternak, O., Rathi, Y., . . . Zafonte, R. (2012). A review of magnetic resonance imaging and diffusion tensor imaging findings in mild traumatic brain injury. *Brain Imaging and Behavior, 6*, 137–192.

Shore, P. M., Berger, R. P., Varma, S., Janesco, K. L., Wisniewski, S. R., Clark, R. S. B., . . . Kochanek, P. M. (2007). Cerebrospinal fluid biomarkers versus Glasgow Coma Scale and Glasgow Outcome Scale in pediatric traumatic brain injury: The role of young age and inflicted injury. *Journal of Neurotrauma, 24*(1), 75–86.

Shores, E. A. (1989). Comparison of the Westmead PTA scale and the Glasgow Coma Scale as predictors of neuropsychological outcome following extremely severe blunt head injury. *Journal of Neurology, Neurosurgery and Psychiatry, 52*(1), 126–127.

Shores, E. A., Marosszeky, J. E., Sandanam, J., & Batchelor, J. (1986). Preliminary validation of a clinical scale for measuring the duration of post-traumatic amnesia. *Medical Journal of Australia, 144*(11), 569–572.

Sigmund, G. A., Tong, K. A., Nickerson, J. P., Wall, C. J., Oyoyo, U., & Ashwal, S. (2007). Multimodality comparison of neuroimaging in pediatric traumatic brain injury. *Pediatric Neurology, 36*(4), 217–226.

Silver, C. H. (2000). Ecological validity of neuropsychological assessment in childhood traumatic brain injury. *Journal of Head Trauma Rehabilitation, 15*(4), 973–988.

Silver, J. (1987). Neuropsychiatric aspects of traumatic brain injury. In R. Hales (Ed.), *The American Psychiatric Press textbook of psychiatry* (pp. 173–184). Washington, DC: American Psychiatric Association.

Sin, N. L., & Lyubomirsky, S. (2009). Enhancing well-being and alleviating depressive symptoms with positive psychology interventions: A practice-friendly meta-analysis. *Journal of Clinical Psychology, 65*(5), 467–487.

Sinnakaruppan, I., Downey, B., & Morrison, S. (2005). Head injury and family carers: A pilot study to investigate an innovative community-based educational programme for family carers and patients. *Brain Injury, 19*(4), 283–308.

Sinopoli, K. J., & Dennis, M. (2012). Inhibitory control after traumatic brain injury in children. *International Journal of Developmental Neuroscience, 30*, 207–215.

Sivan, M., Neumann, V., Kent, R., Stroud, A., & Bhakta, B. B. (2010). Pharmacotherapy for treatment of attention deficits after non-progressive acquired brain injury: A systematic review. *Clinical Rehabilitation, 24*, 10–121.

Skandsen, T., Kvistad, K. A., Solheim, O., Strand, I. H., Folvik, M., & Vik, A. (2010). Prevalence and impact of diffuse axonal injury in patients with moderate and severe head injury: A cohort study of early magnetic resonance imaging findings and 1-year outcome. *Journal of Neurosurgery, 113*, 556–563.

Slater, E. J., & Kohr, M. A. (1989). Academic and intellectual functioning of adolescents with closed head injury. *Journal of Adolescent Research, 4*(3), 371–384.

Slaughter, B., Fann, J. R., & Ehde, D. (2003). Traumatic brain injury in a county jail population: Prevalence, neuropsychological functioning and psychiatric disorders. *Brain Injury, 17*(9), 731–741.

Slifer, K. J. (1996). A video system to help children cooperate with motion control for radiation treatment without sedation. *Journal of Pediatric Oncology Nursing, 13*(2), 91–97.

Slifer, K. J., & Amari, A. (2009). Behavior management for children and adolescents with acquired brain injury. *Developmental Disabilities, 15*, 144–151.

Slifer, K. J., Bucholtz, J. D., & Cataldo, M. D. (1994). Behavioral training of motion control in young children undergoing radiation treatment without sedation. *Journal of Pediatric Oncology Nursing, 11*(2), 55–63.

Slifer, K. J., Koontz, K. L., & Cataldo, M. F. (2002). Operant-contingency-based preparation of children for functional magnetic resonance imaging. *Journal of Applied Behavior Analysis, 35*(2), 191–194.

Sloan, S., Callaway, L., Winkler, D., McKinley, K., Ziino, C., & Anson, K. (2009a). Changes in care and support needs following community-based intervention for individuals with acquired brain injury. *Brain Impairment, 10*(3), 295–306.

Sloan, S., Callaway, L., Winkler, D., McKinley, K., Ziino, C., & Anson, K. (2009b). The community approach to participation: Outcomes following acquired brain injury intervention. *Brain Impairment, 10*(3), 282–294.

Slomine, B. S., Gerring, J. P., Grados, M. A., Vasa, R., Brady, K. D., Christensen, J. R., . . . Denckla, M. B. (2002). Performance on measures of executive function following pediatric traumatic brain injury. *Brain Injury, 16*(9), 759–772.

Slomine, B., & Locascio, G. (2009). Cognitive rehabilitation for children with acquired brain injury. *Developmental Disabilities, 15*, 133–143.

Sohlberg, M., & Mateer, C. (1989). Training use of compensatory memory books: A three-stage behavioral approach. *Journal of Clinical and Experimental Neuropsychology, 11*, 871–891.

Souza, L.G.d.N., Braga, L. W., Filho, G. N., & Dellatolas, G. (2007). Quality-of-life: Child and parent perspectives following severe traumatic brain injury. *Developmental Neurorehabilitation, 10*(1), 35–47.

Spanos, G. K., Wilde, E. A., Bigler, E. D., Cleavinger, H. B., Fearing, M. A., Levin, H. S., . . . Hunter, J. V. (2007). Cerebellar atrophy after moderate-to-severe pediatric traumatic brain injury. *Am J Neuroradiol, 28*(3), 537–542.

Sparrow, S., Balla, D. A., & Cicchetti, D. V. (1984). *Vineland Adaptive Behavior Scales: Interview Edition*. Survey Form Manual. Circle Pines, MN: American Guidance Services.

Stablum, F., Mogentale, C., & Umilta, C. (1996). Executive functioning following mild closed head injury. *Cortex, 32*, 261–278.

Stallings, G. A., Ewing-Cobbs, L., Francis, D. J., & Fletcher, J. M. (1996). Prediction of academic placement after pediatric head injury using neurological, demographic and neuropsychological variables. *Journal of the International Neuropsychological Society, 2*, 39–39.

Stancin, T., Wade, S. L., Walz, N. C., Yeates, K. O., & Taylor, H. G. (2008). Traumatic brain injuries in early childhood: Initial impact on the family. *Journal of Developmental and Behavioral Pediatrics, 29*(4), 253–261.

Statler, K. D. (2006). Pediatric posttraumatic seizures: Epidemiology, putative mechanisms of epileptogenesis and promising investigational progress. *Developmental Neuroscience, 28*, 354–363.

Stierwalt, J.A.G., & Murray, L. L. (2002). Attention impairment following traumatic brain injury. *Seminars in Speech & Language, 23*(2), 129–138.

Stiver, S. L., & Manley, G. T. (2008). Prehospital management of traumatic brain injury. *Neurosurgical Focus, 25*, 1–11.

Stocchetti, N., & Longhi, L. (2010). The race for biomarkers in traumatic brain injury: What science promises and the clinicians still expect. *Critical Care and Medicine, 38*(1), 318–319.

Strauss, E., Sherman, E.M.S., & Spreen, O. (2006). *A compendium of neuropsychological tests: Administration, norms, and commentary* (3rd ed.). New York, NY: Oxford University Press.

Stringer, A.Y. (2011). Ecologically-oriented neurorehabilitation of memory: Robustness of outcome across diagnosis and severity. *Brain Injury, 25*(2), 169–178.

Stuss, D. T., Mateer, C. A., & Sohlberg, M. M. (1994). Innovative approaches to frontal lobe deficits. In M.A.J. Finlayson & S. H. Garner (Eds.), *Brain injury rehabilitation: Clinical considerations* (pp. 212–237). Baltimore, MD: Williams & Wilkins.

Stuss, D. T., Shallice, T., Alexander, M. P., & Picton, T. W. (1995). A multidisciplinary approach to anterior attentional functions. In J. Grafman, K. J. Holyoak, & B. Boller (Eds.), *Structure and function of the human prefrontal cortex* (pp. 191–211). New York, NY: Annals of the New York Academy of Sciences.

Stuss, D. T., & Benson, D. F. (1986). *The frontal lobes.* New York, NY: Raven Press.

Sullivan, C., & Riccio, C. A. (2010). Language functioning and deficits following pediatric traumatic brain injury. *Applied Neuropsychology, 17*, 93–98.

Suskauer, S. J., & Huisman, T. A. (2009). Neuroimaging in pediatric traumatic brain injury: Current and future predictors of functional outcome. *Developmental Disabilities Res Rev, 15*(2), 117–123.

Suzman, K. B., Morris, R. D., Morris, M. K., & Milan, M. A. (1997). Cognitive behavioural remediation of problem solving deficits in children with acquired brain injury. *Journal of Behavior Therapy and Experimental Psychiatry, 28*(3), 203–212.

Swanson, J. O., Vavilala, M. S., Wang, J., Pruthi, S., Fink, J., Jaffe, K. M., . . . Rivara, F. P. (2012). Association of initial CT findings with quality-of-life outcomes for traumatic brain injury in children. *Pediatric Radiology*, doi: 10.1007/s00247–012–2372–8.

Tachtsidis, I., Tisdall, M. M., Pritchard, C., Leung, T. S., Ghosh, A., Elwell, C. E., . . . Smith, M. (2011). Analysis of the changes in the oxidation of brain tissue cytochrome-c-oxidase in traumatic brain injury patients during hypercapnoea: A broadband NIRS study. *Advances in Experimental Medicine and Biology, 701*, 9–14.

Tarazi, R. A., Mahone, E. M., & Zabel, T. A. (2007). Self-care independence in children with neurological disorders: An interactional model of adaptive demands and executive dysfunction. *Rehabilitation Psychology, 52*(2), 196–205.

Tasker, R. C. (2006). Changes in white matter late after severe traumatic brain injury in childhood. *Dev Neurosci, 28*(4–5), 302–308.

Tasker, R. C., Salmond, C. H., Westland, A. G., Pena, A., Gillard, J. H., Sahakian, B. J., . . . Pickard, J. D. (2005). Head circumference and brain and hippocampal volume after severe traumatic brain injury in childhood. *Pediatr Res, 58*(2), 302–308.

Tate, R., Hodgkinson, A., Veerabangsa, A., & Maggiotto, S. (1999). Measuring psychosocial recovery after traumatic brain injury: Psychometric properties of a new scale. *Journal of Head Trauma Rehabilitation, 14*(6), 543–557.

Tate, R. L., McDonald, S., & Lulham, J. M. (1998). Incidence of hospital-treated traumatic brain injury in an Australian community. *Australian and New Zealand Journal of Public Health, 22*, 419–423.

Taylor, H. G., & Alden, J. (1997). Age-related differences in outcomes following childhood brain insults: An introduction and overview. *Journal of the International Neuropsychological Society, 3,* 1–13.

Taylor, H. G., Dietrich, A., Nuss, K., Wright, M., Rusin, J., Bangert, B., . . . Yeates, K. O. (2010). Post-concussive symptoms in children with mild traumatic brain injury. *Neuropsychology, 24*(2), 148–159.

Taylor, H. G., Drotar, D., Wade, S. L., Yeates, K. O., Stancin, T., & Klein, S. (1995). Recovery from traumatic brain injury in children: The importance of the family. In S. H. Broman & M. E. Michel (Eds.), *Traumatic head injury in children* (pp. 188–218). New York, NY: Oxford University Press.

Taylor, H. G., Swartwout, M. D., Yeates, K. O., Walz, N. C., Stancin, T., & Wade, S. L. (2008). Traumatic brain injury in young children: Post-acute effects on cognitive and school readiness skills. *Journal of the International Neuropsychological Society, 14,* 734–745.

Taylor, H. G., Yeates, K. O., Wade, S. L., Drotar, D., Stancin, T., & Burant, C. (2001). Bidirectional child-family influences on outcomes of traumatic brain injury in children. *Journal of the International Neuropsychological Society, 7*(6), 755–767.

Teasdale, G., & Jennett, B. (1974). Assessment of coma and impaired consciousness. *Lancet, 2,* 81–84.

Tellier, A., Marshall, S. C., Wilson, K. G., Smith, A., Perugini, M., & Stiell, I. G. (2009). The heterogeneity of mild traumatic brain injury: Where do we stand? *Brain Injury, 23*(11), 879–887.

Think Quick. (1987). Fremont, CA: The Learning Company.

Thomale, U. W., Graetz, D., Vajkoczy, P., & Sarrafzadeh, A. S. (2010). Severe traumatic brain injury in children—a single center experience regarding therapy and long-term outcome. *Child's Nervous System, 26,* 1563–1573.

Thomson, J. (1995). Rehabilitation of high school-aged individuals with traumatic brain injury through utilization of an attention training program. *Journal of the International Neuropsychological Society, 1*(2), 149.

Thomson, J., & Kerns, K. (2000). Mild traumatic brain injury in children. In S. A. Raskin & C. A. Mateer (Eds.), *Neuropsychological management of mild traumatic brain injury* (pp. 233–251). New York, NY: Oxford University Press.

Timmermans, S. R., & Christensen, B. (1991). The measurement of attention deficits in TBI children and adolescents. *Cognitive Rehabilitation, 9*(4), 26–31.

Timonen, M., Miettunen, J., Hakko, H., Zitting, P., Veijola, J., von Wendt, L., & Rasanen, P. (2002). The association of preceding traumatic brain injury with mental disorders, alcoholism and criminality: The Northern Finland 1966 Birth Cohort Study. *Psychiatry Research, 113*(3), 217–226.

Todd, J. A. (1996). Planning skills in head-injured adolescents and their peers. *Neuropsychological Rehabilitation, 6,* 81–99.

Toledo, E., Lebel, A., Becerra, L., Minster, A., Linnman, C., Maleki, N., . . . Borsook, D. (2012). The young brain and concussion: Imaging as a biomarker for diagnosis and prognosis. *Neuroscience and Biobehavioral Reviews, 36*(6), 1510–1531.

Tong, K. A., Ashwal, S., Holshouser, B. A., Nickerson, J. P., Wall, C. J., Shutter, L. A., . . . Kido, D. (2004). Diffuse axonal injury in children: Clinical correlation with hemorrhagic lesions. *Annals of Neurology, 56*(1), 36–50.

Tong, K. A., Ashwal, S., Holshouser, B. A., Shutter, L. A., Herigault, G., Haacke, E. M., . . . Kido, D. (2003). Hemorrhagic shearing lesions in children and adolescents with post-traumatic diffuse axonal injury: Improved detection and initial results. *Radiology, 227*(2), 332–339.

Tonks, J., Slater, A., Frampton, I., Wall, S. E., Yates, P., & Williams, W. H. (2009). The development of emotion and empathy skills after childhood brain injury. *Developmental Medicine and Child Neurology, 51*(1), 8–16.

Tonks, J., Williams, W. H., Frampton, I., Yates, P., Wall, S. E., & Slater, A. (2007). Reading emotions after childhood brain injury: Case series evidence of dissociation between cognitive abilities and emotional expression processing skills. *Brain Injury, 22*(4), 325–332.

Toussaint, C. P., & Origitano, T. C. (2008). Decompressive craniotomy: Review of induction, outcome, and implication. *Neurosurgery, 18*, 45–53.

Tsaousides, T., & Gordon, W. A. (2009). Cognitive rehabilitation following traumatic brain injury: Assessment to treatment. *Mount Sinai Journal of Medicine, 76*, 173–181.

Tshibanda, L., Vanhaudenhuyse, A., Boly, M., Soddu, A., Bruno, M. A., Moonen, G., . . . Noirhomme, Q. (2009). Neuroimaging after coma. *Neuroradiology, 52*(1), 15–24.

Turkstra, L. S., Dixon, T. M., & Baker, K. K. (2004). Theory of Mind and social beliefs in adolescents. *NeuroRehabilitation, 19*(3), 245–256.

Turkstra, L. S., Williams, W. H., Tonks, J., & Frampton, I. (2008). Measuring social cognition in adolescents: Implications for students with TBI returning to school. *NeuroRehabilitation, 23*, 501–509.

Tyc, V. L., Fairclough, D., Fletcher, B., Leigh, L., & Mulhern, R. K. (1995). Children's distress during magnetic resonance imaging procedures. *Children's Health Care, 24*(1), 5–19.

Umile, E. M., Sandel, M. E., Alavi, A., Terry, C. M., & Plotkin, R. C. (2002). Dynamic imaging in mild traumatic brain injury: Support for the theory of medial temporal vulnerability. *Archives of Physical Medicine and Rehabilitation, 83*(11), 1506–1513.

Vade, A., Sukhani, R., Dolenga, M., & Habisohn-Schuck, C. (1995). Chloral hydrate sedation of children undergoing CT and MR imaging: Safety as judged by American Academy of Pediatrics guidelines. *American Journal of Roentgenology, 165*(4), 905–909.

Vakil, E., Blachstein, H., Rochberg, J., & Vardi, M. (2004). Characterisation of memory impairment following closed head injury in children using the Rey Auditory Verbal Learning Test (RAVLT). *Child Neuropsychology, 10*(2), 57–66.

Valadka, A. B., & Robertson, C. S. (2007). Surgery of cerebral trauma and associated critical care. *Neurosurgery, 61*, SHC203–221.

Valerio, J., & Illes, J. (2011). Ethical implications in neuroimaging in sports concussion. *Journal of Head Trauma Rehabilitation, 27*(3), 216–221.

Van Boven, R. W., Harrington, G. S., Hackney, D. B., Ebel, A., Gauger, G., Bremner, J. D., . . . Weiner, M. W. (2009). Advances in neuroimaging of traumatic brain injury and post-traumatic stress disorder. *Journal of Rehabilitation Research and Development, 46*(6), 717–757.

van den Heuvel, M. P., & Hulshoff Pol, H. E. (2010). Exploring the brain network: A review on resting-state fMRI functional connectivity. *European Neuropsychopharmacology, 20*(8), 519–534.

van Heugten, C. M., Hendriksen, J., Rasquin, S., Dijcks, B., Jaeken, D., & Vles, J. H. (2006). Long-term neuropsychological performance in a cohort of children and adolescents after severe paediatric traumatic brain injury. *Brain Injury, 20*(9), 895–903.

Van Tol, E., Gorter, J. W., DeMatteo, C., & Meester-Delver, A. (2011). Participation outcomes for children with acquired brain injury: A narrative review. *Brain Injury, 25*(13–14), 1279–1287.

van Zomeren, A. H., & Brouwer, W. H. (1994). *Clinical neuropsychology of attention.* New York, NY: Oxford University Press.

Van't Hooft, I., Andersson, K., Bergman, B., Sejersen, J., Von Wendt, L., & Bartfai, A. (2005). Beneficial effect from a cognitive training programme on children with acquired brain injuries demonstrated in a controlled study. *Brain Injury, 19*(7), 511–518.

Van't Hooft, I., Andersson, K., Bergman, B., Sejersen, T., von Wendt, L., & Bartfai, A. (2007). Sustained favourable effects of cognitive training in children with acquired brain injuries. *NeuroRehabilitation, 22,* 109–116.

Van't Hooft, I., & Lindahl Norberg, A. (2010). SMART cognitive training combined with a parental coaching programme for three children treated for medulloblastoma. *Neuro-Rehabilitation, 26,* 105–113.

Varni, J. W., Burwinkle, T.M., Katz, E. R., Meeske, K., & Dickinson, P. (2002). The PedsQL in pediatric cancer: Reliability and validity of the Pediatric Quality of Life Inventory Generic Core Scales, Multidimensional Fatigue Scale, and Cancer Module. *Cancer, 94*(7), 2090–2106.

Varni, J. W., Burwinkle, T. M., & Szer, I. S. (2004). The PedsQL Multidimensional Fatigue Scale in pediatric rheumatology: Reliability and validity. *J Rheumatol, 31*(12), 2494–2500.

Verger, K., Junque, C., Levin, H.S., Jurado, M.A., Perez-Gomez, M., Bartres-Faz, D., . . . Mercader, J.M. (2001). Correlation of atrophy measures on MRI with neuropsychological sequelae in children and adolescents with traumatic brain injury. *Brain Injury, 15*(3), 211–221.

Vogel, A. C., Power, J. D., Petersen, S. E., & Schlaggar, B.L. (2010). Development of the brain's functional network architecture. *Neuropsychology Review, 20*(4), 362–375.

Vu, J. A., Babikian, T., & Asarnow, R. F. (2011). Academic and language outcomes in children after traumatic brain injury: A meta-analysis. *Exceptional Children, 77*(3), 263–281.

Wade, S. L., Carey, J., & Wolfe, C. R. (2006a). An on-line family intervention to reduce parental distress following pediatric brain injury. *Journal of Consulting and Clinical Psychology, 74,* 445–454.

Wade, S., Carey, J., & Wolfe, C. R. (2006b). The efficacy of an online cognitive-behavioral family intervention in improving child behavior and social competence following pediatric brain injury. *Rehabilitation Psychology, 51*(3), 179–189.

Wade, S. L., Cassedy, A., Walz, N. C., Taylor, H. G., Stancin, T., & Yeates, K. O. (2011). The relationship of parental warm responsiveness and negativity to emerging behavior problems following traumatic brain injury in young children. *Developmental Psychology, 47*(1), 119–133.

Wade, S., Chertkoff Walz, N., Carey, J., & Williams, K. M. (2008). Preliminary efficacy of a web-based family problem-solving treatment program for adolescents with traumatic brain injury. *Journal of Head Trauma Rehabilitation, 23*(6), 369–377.

Wade, S., Chertkoff Walz, N., Carey, J. C., & Williams, K. M. (2009). Brief Report: Description of feasibility and satisfaction findings from an innovative online family problem-solving intervention for adolescents following traumatic brain injury. *Journal of Paediatric Psychology, 34*(5), 517–522.

Wade, S., Michaud, L., & Maines Brown, T. (2006). Putting the pieces together. Preliminary efficacy of a family problem-solving intervention for children with traumatic brain injury. *Journal of Head Trauma Rehabilitation, 1,* 57–67.

Wade, S. L., Taylor, H. G., Walz, N. C., Salisbury, S., Stancin, T., Bernard, L. A., . . . Yeates, K. O. (2008). Parent-child interactions during the initial weeks following brain injury in young children. *Rehabilitation Psychology, 53*(2), 180–190.

Wade, S. L., Taylor, H. G., Yeates, K. O., Drotar, D., Stancin, T., Minich, N. M., . . . Schluchter, M. (2006). Long-term parental adaptation and family adaptation following pediatric brain injury. *Journal of Pediatric Psychology, 31,* 1072–1083.

Wade, S. L., Walz, N. C., Carey, J., McMullen, K. M., Cass, J., Mark, E., . . . Yeates, K. (2011). Effect on behavior problems of teen online problem-solving for adolescent traumatic brain injury. *Pediatrics, 128*(4), e1–e7.

Wade, S., Wolfe, C. R., Maines Brown, T., & Pestian, J. P. (2005). Can a web-based family problem-solving intervention work for children with traumatic brain injury? *Rehabilitation Psychology, 50*(4), 337–345.

Walker, P. A., Harting, M. T., Baumgartner, J. E., Fletcher, S., Strobel, N., & Cox, C. S. (2009). Modern approaches to pediatric brain injury therapy. *The Journal of Trauma, 67*, S120–S127.

Walker, W. C., Marwitz, J. H., Kreutzer, J. S., Hart, T., & Novack, T. A. (2006). Occupational categories and return to work after traumatic brain injury: A multicenter study. *Archives of Physical and Medical Rehabilitation, 87*, 1576–1582.

Wallace, B. E., Wagner, A. K., Wagner, E. P., & McDeavitt, J. T. (2001). A history and review of quantitative electroencephalography in traumatic brain injury. *Journal of Head Trauma Rehabilitation, 16*(2), 165–190.

Walz, N. C., Yeates, K. O., Taylor, H. G., Stancin, T., & Wade, S. L. (2009). First-order theory of mind skills shortly after traumatic brain injury in 3- to 5-year-old children. *Developmental Neuropsychology, 34*(4), 507–519.

Walz, N., Yeates, K., Taylor, H., Stancin, T., & Wade, S. (2010). Theory of mind skills 1 year after traumatic brain injury in 6- to 8-year-old children. *Journal of Neuropsychology, 4*, 181–195.

Walz, N. C., Yeates, K. O., Taylor, D. J., Stancin, T., & Wade, S. L. (2011). Emerging narrative discourse skills at 18 months after traumatic brain injury in early childhood. *Journal of Neuropsychology, 6*(2), 143–160.

Ward, H., Shum, D., Dick, B., McKinlay, L., & Baker-Tweney, S. (2004). Intervention study of the effects of paediatric traumatic brain injury on memory. *Brain Injury, 18*(5), 471–495.

Ward, H., Shum, D., McKinlay, L., Baker, S., & Wallace, G. (2009). Prospective memory and pediatric traumatic brain injury: Effects of cognitive demand. *Child Neuropsychology, 13*(3), 219–239.

Ward, H., Shum, D., Wallace, G., & Boon, J. (2002). Pediatric traumatic brain injury and procedural memory. *Journal of Clinical and Experimental Neuropsychology, 24*(4), 458–470.

Warschausky, S. A., Cohen, E. H., Parker, J. G., Levendosky, A. A., & Okun, A. (1997). Social problem-solving skills of children with traumatic brain injury. *Pediatric Rehabilitation, 1*, 77–81.

Watts, D. D., Hanfling, D., Waller, M. A., Gilmore, C., Fakhry, S. M., & Trask, A. L. (2004). An evaluation of the use of guidelines in prehospital management of brain injury. *Prehospital Emergency Care, 8*, 254–261.

Wechsler, D. (1999). *Wechsler Abbreviated Scale of Intelligence* (WASI). San Antonio, TX: Harcourt Assessment.

Wechsler, D. (2002). *The Wechsler Preschool and Primary Scale of Intelligence—Third Edition* (WPSSI-III). London: The Psychological Corporation.

Wechsler, D. (2003). *Manual for the Wechsler Intelligence Scale for Children-IV*. San Antonio, TX: The Psychological Corporation.

Wechsler, D. (2005). *Wechsler Individual Achievement Test—2nd Edition* (WIAT II). London: The Psychological Corporation.

Wells, P., Minnes, P., & Phillips, M. (2009). Predicting social and functional outcomes for individuals sustaining paediatric traumatic brain injury. *Developmental Neurorehabilitation, 12*, 12–23.

West, T. A., & Marion, D. W. (2014). Current recommendations for the diagnosis and treatment of concussion in sport: A comparison of three new guidelines. *Journal of Neurotrauma, 31*(2), 159–168.

Wetherington, C. E., Hooper, S. R., Keenan, H. T., Nocera, M., & Runyun, D. (2010). Parent ratings of behavioral functioning after traumatic brain injury in very young children. *Journal of Pediatric Psychology, 35*(6), 662–671.

Weyandt, L. L., & Willis, W. G. (1994). Executive functions in school aged children: Potential efficacy of tasks in discriminating clinical groups. *Developmental Neuropsychology, 10*(1), 27–38.

Whyte, J. (2009). Directions in brain injury research: From concept to clinical implementation. *Neuropsychological Rehabilitation, 19*(6), 807–823.

Whyte, J., Vaccaro, M., Grieb-Neff, P., & Hart, T. (2002). Psychostimulant use in the rehabilitation of individual with traumatic brain injury. *Journal of Head Trauma Rehabilitation, 17*(4), 284–299.

Wilde, E. A., Bigler, E. D., Hunter, J. V., Fearing, M. A., Scheibel, R. S., Newsome, M. R., . . . Levin, H. S. (2007). Hippocampus, amygdala, and basal ganglia morphometrics in children after moderate-to-severe traumatic brain injury. *Dev Med Child Neurol, 49*(4), 294–299.

Wilde, E. A., Chu, Z., Bigler, E. D., Hunter, J. V., Fearing, M. A., Hanten, G., . . . Levin, H. S. (2006). Diffusion tensor imaging in the corpus callosum in children after moderate to severe traumatic brain injury. *Journal of Neurotrauma, 23*(10), 1412–1426.

Wilde, E. A., Hunter, J. V., & Bigler, E. D. (2012). Pediatric traumatic brain injury: Neuroimaging and neurorehabilitation outcome. *NeuroRehabilitation, 31*(3), 245–260.

Wilde, E. A., Hunter, J. V., Newsome, M. R., Scheibel, R. S., Bigler, E. D., Johnson, J. L., . . . Levin, H. S. (2005). Frontal and temporal morphometric findings on MRI in children after moderate to severe traumatic brain injury. *Journal of Neurotrauma, 22,* 333–344.

Wilde, E. A., McCauley, S. R., Hunter, J. V., Bigler, E. D., Chu, Z., Wang, Z. J., . . . Levin, H. S. (2008). Diffusion tensor imaging of acute mild traumatic brain injury in adolescents. *Neurology, 70*(12), 948–955.

Wilde, E. A., Newsome, M. R., Bigler, E. D., Pertab, J., Merkley, T. L., Hanten, G., . . . Levin, H. S. (2011). Brain imaging correlates of verbal working memory in children following traumatic brain injury. *International Journal of Psychophysiology, 82*(1), 86–96.

Wilke, M., Holland, S. K., Myseros, J. S., Schmithorst, V. J., & Ball, W. S., Jr. (2003). Functional magnetic resonance imaging in pediatrics. *Neuropediatrics, 34*(5), 225–233.

Willer, B. S., Ottenbacher, K. J., & Coad, M. L. (1994). The Community Integration Questionnaire: A comparative examination. *American Journal of Physical Medicine and Rehabilitation, 73*(2), 103–111.

Williams, D., Mehl, R., Yudofsky, S., Adams, D., & Roseman, B. (1982). The effect of propranolol on uncontrolled rage outbursts in children and adolescents with organic brain dysfunction. *Journal of the Academy of Child Psychology, 21,* 129–135.

Williams, S. E. (2007). Amantadine treatment following traumatic brain injury in children. *Brain Injury, 21*(9), 885–889.

Wilson, B. A. (1996). Rehabilitation and management of memory problems. *Acta Neurologica Belgica, 96,* 51–54.

Wilson, B. A. (2000). Compensating for cognitive deficits following brain injury. *Neuropsychology Review, 10,* 233–243.

Wilson, B. A., Alderman, N., Burgess, P. W., Emslie, H., & Evans, J. (1996). *BADS: Behavioural Assessment of the Dysexecutive Syndrome.* London: Thames Valley Test Company.

Wilson, B. A., Baddeley, A., & Evans, J. (1994). Errorless learning in the rehabilitation of memory impaired people. *Neuropsychological Rehabilitation, 4*(3), 307–326.

Wilson, B. A., Emslie, H. C., Quirk, K., & Evans, J. J. (2001). Reducing everyday memory and planning problems by means of a paging system: A randomised control crossover study. *Journal of Neurology, Neurosurgery and Psychiatry, 70*(4), 477–482.

Wilson, J., Wiedmann, K., Hadley, D., Condon, B., Teasdale, G., & Brooks, T. (1988). Early and late magnetic resonance imaging and neuropsychological outcome after head injury. *Journal of Neurology, Neurosurgery and Psychiatry, 51*, 391–396.

Wood, R. (1987). *Brain injury rehabilitation: A neurobehavioural approach.* London: Croon Helm.

Wood, R. L., & Williams, C. (2008). Inability to empathize following traumatic brain injury. *Journal of the International Neuropsychological Society, 14*(2), 289–296.

Woods, D., Catroppa, C., Anderson, V., Matthews, J., Giallo, R., & Barnett, P. (In submission). A family-centred behavioral intervention program for challenging behaviors in children with acquired brain injury: A comparison of two delivery modes. *Journal of Head Trauma Rehabilitation.*

Woods, D., Catroppa, C., Barnett, P., & Anderson, V. (2011). Parental disciplinary practices following acquired brain injury in children. *Developmental Neurorehabilitation, 14*(5), 274–282.

Woods, D., Catroppa, C., Giallo, R., Matthews, J., & Anderson, V. (2012). Feasibility and consumer satisfaction ratings following an intervention for families who have a child with acquired brain injury. *NeuroRehabilitation, 30*, 189–198.

Woods, D., Catroppa, C., Godfrey, C., Giallo, R., Matthews, J., & Anderson, V. (2014). A tele-health intervention for families caring for a child with traumatic brain injury (TBI). *Social Care and Neurodisability, 5*(1), 51–62.

Worley, G., Hoffman, J. M., Paine, S. S., Kalman, S. L., Claerhout, S. J., Boyko, O. B., . . . Oakes, W. J. (1995). 18-fluorodeoxyglucose positron emission tomography in children and adolescents with traumatic brain injury. *Developmental Medicine and Child Neurology, 37*(3), 213–220.

Wozniak, J. R., Krach, L., Ward, E., Mueller, B. A., Muetzel, R., Schnoebelen, S., . . . Lim, K. O. (2007). Neurocognitive and neuroimaging correlates of pediatric traumatic brain injury: A diffusion tensor imaging (DTI) study. *Archives of Clinical Neuropsychology, 22*(5), 555–568.

Wright, I., & Limond, J. (2004). A developmental framework for memory rehabilitation in children. *Pediatric Rehabilitation, 7*(2), 85–96.

Wright, M. J., & Schmitter-Edgecombe, M. (2011). The impact of verbal memory encoding and consolidation deficits during recovery from moderate-to-severe traumatic brain injury. *Journal of Head Trauma Rehabilitation, 26*(3), 182–191.

Wright, R. O., Hu, H., Silverman, E. K., Tsaih, S. W., Schwartz, J., Bellinger, D., . . . Hernandez-Avila, M. (2003). Apolipoprotein E genotype predicts 24-month Bayley Scales Infant Development score. *Pediatric Research, 54*(6), 819–825.

Wu, T. C., Wilde, E. A., Bigler, E. D., Li, X., Merkley, T. L., Yallampalli, R., . . . Levin, H. S. (2010). Longitudinal changes in the corpus callosum following pediatric traumatic brain injury. *Developmental Neuroscience, 32*(5–6), 361–373.

Xu, J., Rasmussen, I., Lagopoulos, J., & Haberg, A. (2007). Diffuse axonal injury in severe traumatic brain injury visualized using high-resolution diffusion tensor imaging. *Journal of Neurosurgery, 24*, 753–765.

Yeates, K. (1999). Closed-head injury. In K. O. Yeates, M. D. Ris, & H. G. Taylor (Eds.), *Pediatric neuropsychology: Research, theory and practice* (pp. 192–218). New York, NY: Guilford Press.

Yeates, K. O. (2010). Mild traumatic brain injury and postconcussive symptoms in children and adolescents. *Journal of the International Neuropsychological Society, 16*(6), 953–960.

Yeates, K. O., Bigler, E. D., Dennis, M., Gerhardt, C. A., Rubin, K. H., Stancin, T., . . . Vannatta, K. (2007). Social outcomes in childhood brain disorder: A heuristic integration of social neuroscience and developmental psychology. *Psychological Bulletin, 133*(3), 535–556.

Yeates, K. O., Blumenstein, E., Patterson, C. M., & Delis, D. C. (1995). Verbal learning and memory following pediatric closed-head injury. *Journal of the International Neuropsychological Society, 1*(1), 78–87.

Yeates, K. O., Kaizer, E., Rusin, J., Bangert, B., Dietrich, A., Nuss, K., . . . Taylor, H. G. (2012). Reliable change in postconcussive symptoms and its functional consequences among children with mild traumatic brain injury. *Archives of Pediatric and Adolescent Medicine, 166,* 615–623.

Yeates, K. O., Ris, M. D., Taylor, H. G., & Pennington, B. F. (Eds.). (2010). *Pediatric neuropsychology: Research, theory, and practice* (2nd ed.). New York, NY: Guilford Press.

Yeates, K. O., Schultz, L. H., & Selman, R. L. (1990). Bridging the gap in child-clinical assessment: Toward the application of social-cognitive developmental theory. *Clinical Psychology Review, 10,* 567–588.

Yeates, K. O., Swift, E. E., Taylor, H. G., Wade, S. L., Drotar, D., Stancin, T., & Minich, N. (2004). Short- and long-term social outcomes following pediatric traumatic brain injury. *Journal of the International Neuropsychological Society, 10,* 412–426.

Yeates, K. O., Taylor, H. G., Chertkoff Walz, N., Stancin, T., & Wade, S. L. (2010). The family environment as a moderator of psychosocial outcomes following traumatic brain injury in young children. *Neuropsychology, 24,* 345–356.

Yeates, K. O., Taylor, H. G., Drotar, D., Wade, S. L., Klein, S., Stancin, T., & Schatschneider, C. (1997). Pre-injury family environment as a determinant of recovery from traumatic brain injuries in school-age children. *Journal of the International Neuropsychological Society, 3,* 617–630.

Yeates, K. O., Taylor, H. G., Rusin, J., Bangert, B., Dietrich, A., Nuss, K., . . . Jones, B. L. (2009). Longitudinal trajectories of postconcussive symptoms in children with mild traumatic brain injuries and their relationship to acute clinical status. *Pediatrics in Review, 123*(3), 735–743.

Yeates, K. O., Taylor, H. G., Wade, S., Drotar, D., Stancin, T., & Minich, N. (2002). A prospective study of short- and long-term neuropsychological outcomes after traumatic brain injury in children. *Neuropsychology, 16*(4), 514–523.

Yeates, K. O., Taylor, H. G., Walz, N. C., Stancin, T., & Wade, S. L. (2010). The family environment as a moderator of psychosocial outcomes following traumatic brain injury in young children. *Neuropsychology, 24*(3), 345–356.

Yeo, R. A., Phillips, J. P., Jung, R. E., Brown, A. J., Campbell, R. C., & Brooks, W. M. (2006). Magnetic resonance spectroscopy detects brain injury and predicts cognitive functioning in children with brain injuries. *Journal of Neurotrauma, 23*(10), 1427–1435.

Ylvisaker, M. (1985). *Head injury rehabilitation: Children and adolescents.* San Diego, CA: College-Hill Press.

Ylvisaker, M., Adelson, P. D., Willandino Braga, L. W., Burnett, S. M., Glang, A., Feeney, T., . . . Todis, B. (2005). Rehabilitation and ongoing support after pediatric TBI: Twenty years of progress. *Journal of Head Trauma Rehabilitation, 20,* 90–104.

Ylvisaker, M., & Feeney, T. (2002). Executive functions, self-regulation and learned optimism in paediatric rehabilitation: A review and implications for intervention. *Pediatric Rehabilitation, 5,* 51–70.

Ylvisaker, M., Szekeres, S. F., & Feeney, T. (1998). Cognitive rehabilitation: Executive functions. In Ylvisaker, M. (Ed.), *Traumatic brain injury rehabilitation: Children and adolescents* (pp. 221–269). Boston, MA: Butterworth-Heinemann.

Ylvisaker, M., Todis, B., Glang, A., Urbanczyk, B., Franklin, C., DePompei, R., . . . Tyler, J. S. (2001). Educating students with TBI: Themes and recommendations. *Journal of Head Trauma and Rehabilitation, 16*(1), 76–93.

Ylvisaker, M., Turkstra, L., Coehlo, C., Yorkston, K., Kennedy, M., Sohlberg, M. M., . . . Avery, J. (2007). Behavioural interventions for children and adults with behaviour disorders after TBI: A systematic review of the evidence. *Brain Injury, 21*(8), 769–805.

Yoganandan, N., Baisden, J. L., Maiman, D. J., Gennarelli, T. A., Guan, Y., Pintar, F. A., . . . Ridella, S. A. (2010). Severe-to-fatal head injuries in motor vehicle impacts. *Acc Anals Prevention, 42,* 1370–1378.

Yuan, W., Holland, S. K., Schmithorst, V. J., Walz, N. C., Cecil, K. M., Jones, B. V., . . . Wade, S. L. (2007). Diffusion tensor MR imaging reveals persistent white matter alteration after traumatic brain injury experienced during early childhood. *American Journal of Neuroradiology, 28*(10), 1919–1925.

INDEX

For Product Safety Concerns and Information please contact our EU
representative GPSR@taylorandfrancis.com
Taylor & Francis Verlag GmbH, Kaufingerstraße 24, 80331 München, Germany

www.ingramcontent.com/pod-product-compliance
Ingram Content Group UK Ltd.
Pitfield, Milton Keynes, MK11 3LW, UK
UKHW021431080625
459435UK00011B/238